CLEAN EATING DIET RECIPES

Clean Eating Meals to Reset Your Body, Metabolism and Weight Loss

(The Ultimate Book Guide to Delicious Recipes)

Brian Hall

Published by Alex Howard

© **Brian Hall**

All Rights Reserved

Clean Eating Diet Recipes: Clean Eating Meals to Reset Your Body, Metabolism and Weight Loss (The Ultimate Book Guide to Delicious Recipes)

ISBN 978-1-990169-03-8

All rights reserved. No part of this guide may be reproduced in any form without permission in writing from the publisher except in the case of brief quotations embodied in critical articles or reviews.

Legal & Disclaimer

The information contained in this book is not designed to replace or take the place of any form of medicine or professional medical advice. The information in this book has been provided for educational and entertainment purposes only.

The information contained in this book has been compiled from sources deemed reliable, and it is accurate to the best of the Author's knowledge; however, the Author cannot guarantee its accuracy and validity and cannot be held liable for any errors or omissions. Changes are periodically made to this book. You must consult your doctor or get professional medical advice before using any of the suggested remedies, techniques, or information in this book.

Table of contents

PART 1 1
INTRODUCTION 2
CHAPTER 1: THE BASICS OF CLEAN EATING 4
CHAPTER 2: RULES OF CLEAN EATING 7
CHAPTER 3: SHOULD YOU FOLLOW THE EAT CLEAN DIET? 10
CHAPTER 4: BENEFITS OF CLEAN EATING 13
CHAPTER 5: UNDERSTANDING THE PRINCIPLES OF CLEAN EATING 15
CHAPTER 6: WHY CHOOSE THE CLEAN EATING LIFESTYLE? 20
CHAPTER 7: THE NEGATIVE EFFECTS OF PROCESSED FOODS 23
CHAPTER 8: SHOPPING SMART AND SEASONAL 27
CHAPTER 9: TIPS & TRICKS TO EATING CLEAN 31
CHAPTER 10: CLEAN EATING MEAL PLAN 38
CHAPTER 11: EATING CLEAN ON THE GO 41
CHAPTER 12: EATING CLEAN FOR WEIGHT LOSS 43
CHAPTER 13: COMMON CLEAN EATING MISTAKES 47
CHAPTER 14: ENERGY-BOOSTING BREAKFAST RECIPES 50

Tortilla with eggs and beans 50
Breakfast taco 51
Egg in Marinara Dressing 53
Baked Mushroom with Baby Spinach 54
Cinnamon and Oats Bowl 55
Coco-Quinoa Burgoo with Strawberry 56
Chia Soleil Pudding 57
Kiwi and Banana Super Bowl 58
Creamy Salmon-Capers 59
Nutty Cookies with a Twist 60
Slow-cooked Sorghum in Pumpkin Purée 61
Rainbow Acai in a Jar 62

CHAPTER 15: SPICE-UP EVERY LUNCH WITH HEALTHY FULLY-LOADED MEALS ... 63

Chile-crusted scallops with cucumber salad ... 63
Hearty Ham Sandwich ... 65
Green Leafy Wraps ... 66
Potato Pizza ... 67
A Taste of the Caribbean ... 67
Shrimp in Collards ... 68
Fruity Detox Drink ... 69
Savory Steak with Salsa ... 70
Asian-style Broccoli Noodles ... 72
Tasty Turkey Tacos ... 73
Crabby-Avocado Salad ... 73

CHAPTER 16: CLEAN EATING DINNER RECIPES UNDER 300 CAL ... 75

Mac n' Cheese Overload ... 75
Lamb Côtelette with Pear Sauce ... 76
Orange Roast Salmon with Rosemary and Thyme ... 77
Seven Veggies with White Fish ... 78
Chicken Dill 'N Dunk Marina ... 79
Irish Ragoût ... 81
Aloha Skewers ... 82
Butterflied grilled chicken with chile-lime rub ... 83

CHAPTER 17: BONUS SMOOTHIES AND DESSERT RECIPES ... 85

Choco cinnamon pudding ... 85
Coconut cranberry cookies ... 85
Hazelnut-Choco Balls ... 86
Banana and Cherry Smoothie ... 87
Rouge Flaxseed Smoothie ... 88

CHAPTER 18: AMAZINGLY CLEAN EATING RECIPES TO START YOUR WEIGHT LOSS ... 89

Mixed Berries Milkshake ... 89
Steak & Veggie Salad ... 90
Creamy Healthy Smoothie ... 91

Pasta & Veggie Salad	92
Chicken & Vegetables Soup	93
Feta Spinach Omelet	94
Green Veggies Soup	95
Noodles & Mixed Vegetables Soup	96
Eggs with Vegetables	97
Tofu & Oats Burgers	98
Tofu with Three Peas	99
Bell Pepper Frittata	100
Chicken Kebabs with Salad	101
Grilled Chicken Thighs	102
Lemony Strawberry French Toasts	103
Shrimp Rolls	104
Veggie Stuffed Chicken Breasts	105
Fruity Oat Muffins	106
Lemony Quinoa & Green Beans	107
Simple Grilled Beef Steak	108
Baked Cherry Pancakes	109
Spinach & Tofu Stir Fry	110
Pork with Bok Choy	111
Quinoa & Date Bowl	111
Broth Braised Cabbage	112
Grilled Lamb Chops & Veggies	113
Nutty Oatmeal	114
Shrimp in Sweet & Sour Sauce	115
Salmon & Veggie Parcel	116

CONCLUSION 117

PART 2 119

Parsley Potatoes	120
Wild Rice Chowder	122
Vegan Bean Burger	123
Chard with Garbanzo Beans and Couscous	125
Garbanzo Curry	126
Vegan Polenta	128
Ginger Stir-Fry with Coconut Rice	129

Avocado Tacos 131
Vegan Style Shepherd's Pie 132
BBQ Tempeh Sandwiches: 134
Vegan Pasta with Pine Nuts 136
Mediterranean Zucchini 137
Pumpkin-Apple Curry 138
Garlic-Ginger Tofu 140
Baked Potato with Lentils 141
Vegan Mac and No-Cheese 143
Soba Noodles 144
Spicy Potato Curry 145
Quinoa Chard Pilaf 147
Tofu Broccoli Quiche 148
Lentil and Veggies 150
Grilled Tomato-Balsamic Veggies with Couscous 152
Tempeh Fajitas 153
Lentil, Kale, and Red Onion Pasta 154
Teriyaki Tofu with Pineapple 155
Tofu and Red Bell Peppers with Spicy Peanut Sauce 156
Toasted Almond and Quinoa Salad 158
Vegan Chili 159

ONE-POT MARRAKESH STEW 162

Crispy Sesame Tofu and Broccoli 164
Stuffed Sweet Potatoes 165
Tofu Kebabs with Cilantro Dressing 166
Four-Grain Vegan Salad 167
Barley with Winter Greens Pesto 169
Cajun Style Tempeh Po' Boy 170
Celery Root Soup 172
Garbanzo Cakes with Mashed Avocado 174

VEGAN PAELLA 176

Spicy Quinoa with Edamame 178
Avocado Pasta with Blackened Veggies 179
Black-eyed Peas with Collard Greens and Turnips 180

Vegan Black Bean Quesadillas 182
Stuffed Red Bell Pepper 183
Couscous with Olives and Sun-dried Tomatoes 184
Braised White Beans and Chard 187
Miso Soup with Napa Cabbage 189

Part 1

Introduction

In recent years, there has been a surge of diet plans and programs. This is in response to the increasing consciousness of people regarding their weight and overall health. This increase in the number of "healthy" eating plans and programs is also out of the escalating incidence of heart problems, diabetes, and other lifestyle diseases. One of the programs that is making a name for itself in the health and wellness industry is the Clean Eating program.

What Is Clean Eating?

The Clean Eating program doesn't literally pertain to the cleanliness of the food. It focuses more on how the food is prepared. In contrast with other eating plans out there, this program is not made specifically for people who want simply to lose weight. In fact, it makes a stand that it isn't a diet but rather a lifestyle, a way of life. The program is all about eating food in its most natural form. This means eating whole, unrefined or unprocessed food. Unprocessed foods are those that are with little or no preservatives at all.

Clean Eating is all about the consumption of whole foods like fruits, vegetables, lean meats, healthy fats, and complex carbohydrates. The basic idea of Clean Eating is not new. The principle behind this program is rooted in the natural health movement in the 1960s. This health movement focused on the whole food approach to eating. It also promoted the consumption of unprocessed food.

Although the idea behind this eating program has been around for quite some time now, it wasn't widely known until Tosca Reno published a series of Clean Eating cookbooks. Reno is a Canadian fitness model who popularized this eating program. The principle is still the same as it was with the natural health movement in the 1960s.

What It Is

The Clean Eating program is for people who want to make intelligent and healthier choices, who want to get fit, who want to feel better, and who want to limit their intake of processed food. Because this eating program is aimed towards the consumption of foods at their most natural, unprocessed form, taking part in it will enable your body to function at its best and, consequently, will make you feel fantastic and full of energy. This is far from the fad diets that have been lurking around, most of which make you feel lethargic, deprived, and hungry.

What It Is Not

If you're looking for another fad diet, then the Clean Eating program is not for you. The proponents of the program made it clear that this is not a diet but more of a way of life. If you're overweight, this program can help you lose those excess pounds. It can also help those who have problems in gaining weight.

Unlike other eating programs that you can find out there, it doesn't require you to starve yourself or make you count anything like calories, points, carbs, grams, and fat. You don't have to buy pre-packaged or pre-portioned food, and it doesn't require you to take pills or special potions. What this eating program calls for is the choice of choosing whole and natural foods.

Chapter 1: The Basics of Clean Eating

If you've been keen about the latest trend in health lately, then you've probably heard about Clean Eating. In contrast to what other people believe, Clean Eating is not a diet. This is a lifestyle choice as its proponents suggests. Unlike fad diets, Clean Eating won't promise that you'll lose any excess pounds. It doesn't even promote calorie or point counting. What it does instead is encourage healthy eating.

To get started with the Clean Eating program, it is important to get to know the basics of this program:

1. Fruits and Vegetables

Fruits and vegetables are important elements of this eating program. While it is not the center of the Clean Eating program, the consumption of these foods is a basic part of it. Because fruits and vegetables are rich in vitamins and minerals, the American Cancer Society promotes the consumption of five servings of these foods a day.

Fruits and vegetables have cleansing and detoxifying properties. For instance, kale has detoxifying properties while celery eliminates excess fluids in the body. Apples also have healing compounds that get rid of carcinogenic toxins in the body. Lemons can eliminate putrefactive bacteria and mucous buildup in the intestines.

2. Lean Proteins

Other than fruits and vegetables, the Clean Eating program also advocates a diet comprised of lean proteins. This includes plant-based proteins that are low in fat and high in fiber. Examples of plant-based proteins include beans, legumes, tofu, and other soy-based products. Other sources of lean proteins include white meat poultry, fish, and lean cuts of beef.

Lean proteins are excellent sources of B vitamins, such as niacin and riboflavin, iron, magnesium, zinc, and vitamins E and C. B vitamins can help you raise your energy levels and improve nervous system function. Zinc, on the other hand, can help the immune system function normally.

3. Whole Grains

Because Clean Eating is all about eating foods in their most basic form, this includes the presence of whole grains. Whole grains are unprocessed foods that have a higher concentration of fiber and protein than their processed counterpart. Whole grains are good sources of energy but are low in saturated fat. Examples of whole grains are bread, oatmeal, wheat germ, flaxseed, brown rice, and whole wheat pasta.

Whole grains are extremely popular in many dietary programs, and this is because it can help a dieter maintain weight and improve his health. According to studies, whole grains can help carotid arteries become healthier and reduce the risk of a variety of medical conditions such as colorectal cancer, heart problems, gum disease, and hypertension.

4. Water

Other than healthy and natural food sources, another important part of Clean Eating is water. Sufficient intake of water is promoted by this eating program. Unlike soda and other sugar-laden drinks, water has zero calories and doesn't contain any sugar. It helps regulate the body's functions and aids in improving one's metabolism. An intake of 8 glasses or more of water per day is advised.

Drinking the recommended amount of water per day can help you maintain the balance of fluids in your body. It can help maintain the right body temperature as well as improve circulation and transportation of nutrients.

5. Healthy Snacks

Forget about cookies, chips, and cakes. Clean Eating is not about those snacks since they are high in saturated fat. In this eating program, food options for snacks are still in line with the program's principle. Instead of pastries that are high in fat and drinks which are overloaded with sugar, the Clean Eating program promotes healthy snacks such as fruits, nuts, vegetables, whole grain crackers, and low-fat milk or yogurt.

Don't be confused with what to and what not to eat. If you know the principle of Clean Eating by heart, then you don't have to fret over food choices. You'll know that to be healthy you just have to choose foods existing in their most natural form.

Chapter 2: Rules of Clean Eating

If you haven't tried any form of eating program before, the principle of Clean Eating might seem overwhelming for you. It may sound complex, but looking at its core principle, you will find out that it's very simple. Incorporating the Clean Eating program into your regular lifestyle can be easy. To help you get started with it, here are the rules of Clean Eating:

1. Focus on fresh produce

These include fruits and vegetables grown organically if possible. Aside from needed vitamins and minerals, fruits and vegetables also provide you with dietary fiber, needed for flushing out waste and toxins from your body. This natural product can help you feel healthier and better.

Although you can still get nutrients by consuming health-promoting supplements, doing it will make you feel hungrier and deprived. It will make you cheat and resort to eating unhealthy foods impulsively just to satisfy your hunger. Find the best-tasting fruits and vegetables that are in season and make it a habit to consume them.

2. Avoid processed foods

Processed foods are often loaded with artificial flavoring, sodium, sugar and saturated fats. While some of these substances help in prolonging the food's shelf life and improve their palatability, they won't do anything good for your health. Clean Eating keeps you from consuming this kind of food product. You should also avoid consumption of refined foods such as white bread as they are less healthy options.

The processed foods that you should avoid include canned foods as they have huge amounts of fat and sodium. You should also avoid eating pasta meals that are not made of whole grains. You also should not eat packaged snack foods such as chips, frozen dinners which are high in sodium, sugary breakfast cereals, processed meats, and boxed meal mixes.

3. Eat 5–6 meals in a day

Several studies have already been conducted regarding the benefits of having more than 3 meals a day. According to these studies, having small, frequent meals in a day could help in maintaining a healthy weight and even promote weight loss for those who are overweight. This is because eating more than three times a day could help you curb your cravings. However, this should be done with certain considerations – one of which is to make sure that every meal is healthy. So, it would be a no-no to eat sugar- and salt-laden meals.

4. Have a balanced meal

What sets the Clean Eating program from other eating programs out there is that it focuses more on nutrition than the idea of making you lose weight. One of the key rules of Clean Eating is to eat a balanced meal on a daily basis. It won't restrict you from carbohydrates or fats. Instead, it motivates you to choose healthier alternatives like choosing complex over simple carbs and healthy fats as opposed to trans fats. You can consume unsaturated fats such as omega-3 and omega-6 fatty acids.

5. Drink more water

The importance of a sufficient intake of water has been stressed by health gurus for decades now. Aside from hydrating your body, water helps in maintaining normal body processes. Drinking sufficient amounts of water is also necessary for those who are working out. According to research, water plays a significant role in the growth of muscles and the prevention of catabolism.

6. Check the ingredients

Learn to read food labels. Avoid food products with ingredients that you can't read. If it bears ingredients that you can hardly read, pronounce, or understand, then it's better to ditch that food. Clean Eating is all about food simplicity, and this means that you need to consume foods that have minimal or no additives. It is also best that you avoid purchasing products that contain 5 to 6 ingredients or more. Products with a long list of ingredients are often unhealthy and overprocessed.

7. Approach each meal as part of your lifestyle

One of the best things about the Clean Eating program is that it's sustainable. This means that you can do it for life, regardless of whether or not you want to lose weight. If you want to be part of this revolutionary eating program, then be prepared to change your approach to food. Try to consider clean eating as something that you can practice for the rest of your life.

8. Prioritize the nutrients

Your clean-eating plan should focus more on nutrients than calories. Of course, it is important to measure your caloric intake. However, it is not becoming thin that makes you healthy but having the right body weight. You can achieve and maintain the right weight if you focus on nourishing your body with the right amount of nutrients it needs. Satisfying your nutritional needs can positively affect your weight and health.

You should stop thinking about calories or point counting as there is no need to do so here. All that you are required to do is to settle with natural and healthy produce and consider eating them regularly.

Chapter 3: Should You Follow the Eat Clean Diet?

Clean Eating has become synonymous with healthy eating. This is thanks to the series of Clean Eating books released by Tosca Reno, a bestselling author, columnist, motivational speaker, and consultant. With the increasing popularity of this eating program comes the question, "Will it work for everybody?"

This skepticism is totally understandable. Although the advocates of this eating program stress that it isn't a diet, history has shown that not all people respond the same way to diets or eating programs. Some have a positive response, while there are also those who have minimal or no favorable response at all.

How the Eat Clean Diet Works

The Eat Clean diet works through its promotion of natural produce and whole grain products, combined with physical activity and calorie-controlled meals. It involves eating foods in their natural state and taste. When the body takes high quality food, it apparently becomes stronger and healthier. If it is fuelled with low-grade food, it will become weak and more susceptible to illnesses. This diet ensures that your body will only be taking foods that can make your internal organs work at their best. Since these foods are rich in nutrients and do not contain harmful substances, your body will only receive the vitamins and minerals it needs.

This eating program is comprised of the following key points: 80% food, 10% exercise, and 10% genes.

Experts' Reviews

There are good points to this natural and pure approach to healthy eating. The program's goal is to promote the consumption of food items like whole grain products, fruits, vegetables, complex carbohydrates, healthy fats, and lean protein. However, just like other programs, it isn't perfect. Some experts have criticized certain aspects of this program.

According to Roberta Anding, MS, RD, the spokeswoman of American Dietetic Association, you can follow the basic rules and use its meal suggestions but skip the nutrition advice from the program. Following the program's nutrition and supplement advice could lead to certain deficiencies. Anding added that there are studies that prove that small amounts of alcohol, which is discouraged in this program, could be helpful as it can be cardio-protective. She further stresses that small amounts of saturated fat are unavoidable and not totally harmful to one's health.

Another nutrition expert, Priya Kathpal, says the same thing about the program. According to Kathpal, following a program without an expert's guidance could lead to deficiencies. For her, it's also not feasible to always have organic produce since the availability of organically grown fruits and vegetables vary from one place to another. This program, in her opinion, is costly since organically grown products cost more than those that are not.

Other issues being raised in this program is its restrictive structure, which can also raise issues on its sustainability. Programs like the Eat Clean diet can be difficult to follow in the long run.

Why Follow the Diet?

The expert's review stated that nutritional deficiencies may take place while following this diet. However, studies have shown that the deficiencies only take place when the dieter does not follow a nutritionally balanced meal plan.

As a matter of fact, nutritional deficiencies are more prevalent to people who are following other diet programs. Other dietary programs that don't discourage the consumption of processed foods are more likely to cause nutritional deficiencies. Most processed products go through rigorous treatments before being sold in the market. According to several studies, extensive processing does not just add harmful substance but also removes the nutrients contained in foods. Some diet experts even believe in the efficiency of the program when it comes to weight loss and health improvement.

Do You Want to Be Leaner and Healthier?

If you are aiming at becoming leaner and healthier, then this diet is a good choice. It recommends foods that are rich in antioxidants, vitamins, fiber, and healthy fats. These foods are also preservative-free, which makes them healthier options. Plenty of dieters have already experienced overall improvement of their health condition by following the diet.

Eating small meals frequently can help your reduce cravings and hunger. You won't also gain extra pounds because you will consume less fat and sugar. With these, you can lose 3 pounds a week while practicing the diet. These are excess and unwanted fats that you can get rid of while following this dietary program. Once you achieve the body and weight that suits you, you will be able to maintain it by continuing the diet.

Is It Right for You?

Because you have the freedom to choose your own food, the Eat Clean diet is relatively safe for those who are on a vegan diet or are vegetarians, as well as those with allergies, and/or those with certain dietary restrictions. Diabetics and people with special health considerations should consult their physician for some adjustments.

You can make the easiest transformation from being sluggish to being energetic by simply eating clean. Fitness professionals even find the diet a brilliant way to change a person eating habits on a daily basis.

Chapter 4: Benefits of clean eating

Weight loss

One of the biggest benefits of eating clean is weight loss. If you clean up your day, you will naturally lose weight and become slimmer. This will not only leave you looking better, but feeling better too. And there are numerous benefits that losing just 10lbs has on the body, including lower blood pressure, lower cholesterol, less risk of heart disease, less stress on the joints and less stress on the body's major organs.

Better mood

Research has shown that a higher consumption of fruit and vegetables results in increased energy, calmness and greater feelings of overall happiness. It was also noted that the effects of an elevated mood were not just present on the days when the higher consumption of healthy produce was consumed, but also carried over through to the following day.

Sounder night's sleep

Clean eating doesn't just have an effect on your waistline, but consuming the right foods can help aid a good night's sleep. Foods than have been linked to better slumber include, fish, whole grains, nuts and dark leafy greens. Research has also suggested that consuming two pieces of kiwi fruit before going to bed can help you drop off to sleep faster and sleep sounder. In a nutshell, a better diet leads to better sleep.

Enhanced workouts

A clean diet can enable you to have better workouts. Eating a healthy diet will not only provide you with the energy needed to blast through your workouts, but a clean diet will also help the body recover from that strenuous workout after. Healthy foods are known to build muscle, aid recovery and improve endurance.

Radiant glowing skin

According to research, eating clean will leave you radiating with a natural glow. Eating more fruits and vegetables will lead to a smoother, clearer complexion and help soften the skin. So a healthy diet does not just work wonders on the inside, but on the outside too.

Improved cognitive function

For a long time the Mediterranean diet has been heralded as a great example for optimal health. The fundamentals of the Mediterranean diet consist of fruits, vegetables, fish, beans, olive oil, avocado, whole grains, nuts and seeds, with a lower consumption of dairy products, fatty meats, refined grains and added sugars. Research has shown that those that consistently adhere to a Mediterranean style diet were less likely to have brain infarcts – small areas of dead tissue on the brain that are linked to cognitive disorders.

Chapter 5: Understanding The Principles of Clean Eating

You have now gathered a decent idea on what clean eating is all about, so let us look at a few principles that will help you with eating healthy. You will need to keep these principles in mind before you jump on board with clean eating.

Natural food over processed food

If you purchase food from the supermarket and find that you are picking up products that come out of a bag, can, or even a box, remind yourself that these foods are definitely processed. However, you may think to yourself that the frozen vegetables are not processed, so why choose frozen vegetables instead of fresh produce? When you consume fresh food, you will be able to ensure that you have great health for a very long time. It is always good to consume fresh and crisp food if you are looking at keeping yourself healthy. If you find that you are feeling good on the inside it will reflect on the outside.

Prefer unrefined food

This is a fact that everybody needs to remember! Make sure that you consume your share of wheat, rice, barley, millets and quinoa whenever you can! It is always good to consume food that gives you protein – make sure that the food is not refined! If you love sweetened food, make sure that you consume maple syrup or even honey instead of downing spoons of sugar. Always choose these foods over boxed foods since they are the best for your health.

Always consume a balanced meal

When you are preparing a meal for yourself, you have to ensure that you have not broken the contents of the meal down. Do not tell yourself that you need proteins and carbohydrates right before a workout since this does not help your body. You will have to include every nutrient that you need in one meal a day! You will have to avoid depriving your body of these nutrients simply because of a certain a schedule or diet you used to follow.

Keep an eye on sugar and fat

The fat we are discussing about here is trans-fat which is extremely and terribly bad for your body. These fats find their homes in your arteries and conveniently block them causing millions of heart diseases. If you consume salt and sugar in the right amounts you would not be harming your body. But, too much of these ingredients would only lead to numerous health issues that you would never want to be associated with ever!

Always understand your body's needs

Every human is different from the next. The way your body is built is definitely different from the way mine is built. Therefore, it is difficult to tell you to stick to a diet that I may have tried since that may not work for you! You have to consume three meals a day and will need to ensure that you have included every group of food into those meals. The minute you begin to skip meals, your body begins to starve itself and will use up the fat in your body. This is good news but what you have forgotten is that the next time you eat food, it all gets stored as fat in your body! You could also consume healthy snacks in between if that is what your body needs! Make sure that you consume a salad or fruit.

Always exercise!

This is something that you will definitely need to do. You will not have to work out in the gym for hours together. You just need to ensure that you continue to move. If you are watching the television and the advertisements have begun, go for a walk around the living room. Make sure that you incorporate as much exercise as possible. There are countless apps for smart phones and other short 5 minute workout programs you can include in your day to day life.

Always shop smart

When you have entered the supermarket, what aisle do you walk up to first? You will walk up to the aisles where you have seen the numerous boxes with all the lovely food stored in them. You put the fresh produce out of your mind and continue to shop for these packaged items! The next time you enter a supermarket, walk up to the fresh produce first and pick the ingredients you need before you walk down the other aisles.

No added sugar

This is a principle that every human being has to follow! You will need to stop consuming excessive amounts of sugar. You will only be feeding your body with calories that do nothing to keep you healthy. Food in the natural form contains the required amounts of sugar. You could consume fruits or even a few vegetables to obtain the sugar you want. Ensure that you do not consume cold fruit juices or soda since they are filled to their brim with sugar. Just take a look at the amount of sugar in a can of soda. You will find yourself loving natural foods when you have warmed up to the idea mentioned above. You may find that not consuming as much sugar as normal will decrease your energy levels, but that is okay! The reason why is that your body will need to go through a temporary transitional period in which your body is not so heavily reliant on artificial energy through the means of consuming sugar. Once this transitional period has passed, you will have constant real and healthy energy!

Drink lots of water

You have been told that you need to consume close to eight or ten glasses of water and this is with great reason. There are reasons behind this. The first is that you have to keep your body hydrated since your muscles will be able to respond faster and you will also be able to continue to the work out with ease. The second is that the organs in your body will begin to function in the normal way. The final reason is that you always confuse your thirst with hunger!

Always sit down to eat

Every human being has become very busy these days. They do not have the time to sit down and consume their meal since they are always rushing out of the house in order to get to work on time. Other times you consume your dinner in front of the television. You will find that you will consume too much food that may also include junk. You have to stop this and will need to start making sure that you make every meal a special affair. You will need to set the table out and also ensure that you serve each morsel with care. You could invite friends over and also have your family sitting with you at the table. You will find that you will be able to consume a great home cooked meal.

Are you scared of the flour used in desserts?

You could definitely eat that lovely pastry, the mouthwatering pie, and the lovely cake just by substituting the flour with a healthier version of the flour! You could definitely use millet flour or even almond flour instead of the all – purpose flour when you are baking at home. You will find that the final product is not that different from the original recipe and the advantage here is that you will be able to eat your favorite food in its healthiest form.

Always consume food you understand

When you are looking at the boxes you have purchased, have you made the effort to read the list of ingredients that have been mentioned at the back of the box? Do you understand every ingredient that has been mentioned? Are there certain items that you cannot read at all? Can you pronounce every ingredient? It is best if you do not consume such processed foods filled with preservatives. You could always choose to stick to food that you have a great knowledge of. If you find that the food you want to eat comes in a box, you will need to chuck it. Always try to use food that you can read and pronounce. The food could be exotic but this does not mean it is good for your health. Always consume whole food!

Nutrition is more important than calories

Every person in the world has become very conscious of the food that he or she consumes. It is true that people need to control their caloric intake, but this does not mean they cut it out of their diet. The calories are needed by your body in order to help it function. You need to focus on the nutritional value of the food you consume and stop worrying about the calories. Your body is more intelligent than you know and can always differentiate between good and bad calories.

Chapter 6: Why Choose the Clean Eating Lifestyle?

Eating a clean and unprocessed diet is first and foremost for your overall health. Weight loss is just an added bonus. You must enter into this decision with the mentality that you are doing this for the big picture because getting into a state of better health is paramount. We come equipped with only one ephemeral vessel to carry us throughout our years and that cliché' phrase, "You are what you eat" remains true. The food we choose fuels these wondrous machines of ours. In order to best care for ourselves and ensure a long and healthy life, we must become more mindful of our eating habits.

We have discussed the many benefits of what I call a lifestyle because it requires you to change your outlook and not just your grocery list. Now, we will touch on the results you will experience by using this knowledge over any fad diet. Dr. Layne Norton claims that most diets fail due to lack of consistency and an inability to adapt the lifestyle necessary for continuance on your path. His research has also found that within a year, 80% of dieters will gain back the weight they had lost and a quarter of those eventually gain more weight. This yo-yo effect of crash dieting is extremely detrimental to your health, motivation and progress.

Adopting a clean lifestyle encourages the intake of fruits, vegetables, lean meats, nuts, seeds, healthy grains and fats. It also promotes exercise and restricts additives and preservatives commonly found in most processed foods. Chowing down on nuts like almonds or walnuts, for example, can lower your cholesterol and thereby greatly reducing the risk of heart disease. These, as well as olive oil, avocados, and fatty fish like salmon, all have something in common. They contain unsaturated fats. Monounsaturated and polyunsaturated fats – including the famed omega 3 and omega 6 – are essential fatty acids that your body can't make on its own. Whole grain fiber and protein from nuts, legumes and lean meats are digested slowly and serve as a sustainable energy source that will keep you fuller for longer periods of time. And among other benefits, plant foods contain the high probiotic and enzyme content essential for a healthy intestinal ecology. Thriving gut flora enables proper nutrient absorption and disposal of waste.

A study published in the British Journal of Health Psychology suggested that young adults who observed a clean eating lifestyle experienced a greater "flourishing", meaning they were happier, more positive, creative, and curious. Another study, found in the Australian and New Zealand Journal of Psychiatry, has found a correlation in patients who experienced psychosis and their intake of fruits and vegetables. There are countless other social experiments and studies which point to an overall feeling of happiness and tranquility associated with clean eating habits. When we understand what our bodies need to thrive and provide them with such they will in turn take care of us!

Have you ever had trouble falling asleep or staying asleep? Can you not seem to relax or clear your mind? Well, you are not alone. Over 50 million Americans claim they do not get enough sleep. Modifying your diet to include fish such as salmon, halibut, and tuna can boost vitamin B which is needed to make Melatonin, the sleep-inducing hormone. I would bet that you never thought of carb loading to induce sleep, either. Well, in one study conducted by the American Journal of Clinical Nutrition, participants who consumed high glycemic index (GI) jasmine rice at dinner fell asleep faster than those who had a meal prepared with lower GI long-grain rice. This could be attributed to the greater amount of insulin which jump started the production of tryptophan, another sleep-inducing chemical.

Whatever your reason for taking up the cause of caring for your body might be, whether it's weight loss, better sleep, improved brain and gut health, immune boost, high cholesterol, cancer treatment, or even a general state of happiness and well-being, the importance of eating for your health is obvious and the time is now.

Chapter 7: The Negative Effects of Processed Foods

An epidemic is currently sweeping this nation with over half of Americans classified as either overweight or obese. Ranking among the lowest of industrialized nations in terms of life expectancy, Americans spend on average about $1,200 each year on fast food. Monetary concerns aside, the negative health effects of processed foods are staggering. Foods can be considered processed through a number of alterations ranging from chemical fillers to just adding heat during cooking. Observing a clean eating lifestyle, you would want to stay as close to the foods whole and natural state as possible. The exception would be a process - such as cooking or dehydrating at home - that doesn't add harmful chemicals into the mix. When foods start receiving chemical fillers, additives, and preservatives that is when we cross over into more dangerous territory. Junk foods are comprised of anything that contain hydrogenated fats, chemicals, nitrates, preservatives, or a high refined sugar content. These processed options have something in common; the cost of digesting, absorbing, and eliminating these non-foods is far greater than any nutritional and caloric benefit they may offer.

The ancient art of food preservation such as canning, salting, fermentation, and sun-drying are almost extinct in the modern world of mass production. Today, there are thousands of additives and chemicals used by food companies. Not all of which are bad such as the addition of calcium or vitamins. Many of these, however, can wreak havoc on our bodies.

Nitrates are chemicals used to preserve and cure certain meats and have been associated with cancer, asthma, nausea, and headaches. Sulfur dioxide is another toxic preservative that is used in dried fruit and molasses and also prevents brown spots on peeled fresh food like apples. The application of this chemical snuffs out the vitamin B content of these foods and often hides telltale signs of inferior produce. When you hear that antioxidants may be used to preserve certain foods, you would probably think, "Great! Antioxidants are good for the body, right?" Well, not always. Antioxidants such as BHA (butylated hydroxyanisole) and BHA (butylated hydroxytoluene) are two of the most controversial and widely used examples. The results of animal testing were so disturbing, that a number of countries have significantly restricted their use or banned them altogether. Some scientists have found correlations between these additives and hyperactivity disorder, behavioral problems, allergic reactions, cancer, and neurological damage. Despite these findings, the United States has not put any limitations on companies who use these antioxidants. The prevalence of BHA and BHT in food products has actually increased in the U.S.

Artificial food dyes are another additive that food companies use in everything from orange rinds, to chicken feed in order to produce a more yellow yolk. Blue #1 was found to cause kidney tumors in mice, according to an unpublished study concerning the effects of dyes on animal subjects. Blue #2, commonly found in colored beverages, candies, and pet food was found to significantly increase the incidence of brain gliomas and other tumors in male rats. Citrus red #2 is the dye used to enhance the color of orange skins and also caused tumors in rodents. Recognized in 1990 as a thyroid carcinogen, red #3 is added to sausage casings, maraschino cherries, and candies. Red #40 is widely consumed and has been said to accelerate immune system tumors in mice. Found in baked goods, dessert powders, candies, cereals, and cosmetics, "Allura Red" has also been linked to hyperactivity in children. Yellow #5 and yellow #6 have both been studied in connection with hypersensitivity and hyperactivity in children and adrenal tumors in rodents. These two are commonly found in products such as gelatin desserts, candies, soda, and cosmetics.

With the frighteningly high prevalence of Autism and hyperactivity disorders observed in American children recently, one cannot help but to connect the dots from the harmful chemicals added to food during processing to an exponential increase in these diseases. According to the CDC as of 2011, approximately 11% of children – 6.4 million – have been diagnosed with ADHD. The percentage of children with a hyperactivity diagnosis has significantly increased from 7.8% in 2003. Rates of ADHD diagnoses increased on an average of 3% per year from 1997-2006 and approximately 5% per year from 2003-2011. As well as these hyperactivity disorders, Autism spectrum disorders have consistently been on the rise parallel with increased use of additives in mass produced foods. Records from the CDC have shown that ASD is on the rise from 1 in 150 in 2000 to 1 in 68 as of 2012. Considering the calculation of growth, diagnoses have likely soared to 1 in 50 or less in 2015.

Artificial sweeteners have been the subject of much scrutiny over the years. New alternatives come and go. Most notably, saccharine and aspartame. Saccharine was found to increase the incidence of bladder cancer in animals and companies that still use this product have been required to include warning information on the label. Aspartame is one of the most common artificial sweetener used today. Countless studies have been conducted about the safety of aspartame and most were inconclusive or chalked up to coincidence and other variables. Consumers have reported headaches, dizziness, digestive symptoms and mood swings as well as more serious health issues like Alzheimer's, birth defects, diabetes, hyperactivity and attention deficit disorders, Parkinson's disease, lupus, multiple sclerosis and seizures. However, studies on these effects have proved inconclusive as well. The most common additive used by the food industry are artificial flavorings with over 2000 different formulations currently in use. These chemicals are not required to be listed though some have been linked to allergic and behavioral reactions.

The refining process of wheat and other grains strips away the outer husk, leaving a refined starch which is easily broken down into sugar. This allows the starch to be absorbed into the bloodstream quickly which causes a rise in glucose levels and leads to obesity. Purchasing whole grains will ensure that the fibrous bran remains intact so that they are absorbed into the bloodstream more slowly. When the wheat germ and bran are removed during the milling process, so are the majority of key nutrients found in wheat. 50-93% of wheat's vitamin E, unsaturated fats, magnesium, zinc, chromium, manganese, calcium, phosphorous, potassium, iron, riboflavin, thiamin, niacin, and cobalt are lost during refining.

Chapter 8: Shopping Smart and Seasonal

Grocery shopping with clean eating in mind does not have to be daunting. With some knowledge and planning, you can become as well-versed and focused as a contestant on supermarket sweep! My number one advice when taking on the task of meal planning and grocery shopping for a clean diet is to think ahead. Sit down once a week and consider what you would like to eat. This book contains a few recipes to get you started. I also find that checking my local sale paper beforehand helps me to find a few deals and make the trip a bit easier on my bank account. As well as benefitting from sale papers and coupons, familiarize yourself with the harvest times of your favorite produce. Buying a mango when they are out of season will set you back almost double – sometimes more – than when they are in season. As well as the price, fruits and vegetables taste the best when they are not forced out of season. Ever eaten a peach so juicy and ripe that unintentionally utter slurping noises and somehow end up with your entire arm covered in sweet sticky nectar? Compare that to the misfortune of purchasing a peach during the fall. You bite into it only to experience a disappointing texture and less than desirable flavor. If the clean eating diet had a motto it would be, "Nature Knows Best." Gain some knowledge about crops that are grown in your area and their harvest times. Buying fresh, local, in season produce is a win-win. The items you purchase will undoubtedly be delicious and cost effective. You will also be supporting your local economy!

Now that you have planned your meals for the week and skimmed your sale paper, you are ready to take on the big box giants. Whenever possible, visit your local farmers market or you-pick field. Taking advantage of local produce, especially local honey, is a healthful and community-minded way to do your shopping. When you do venture into your supermarket, remember this major piece of advice: Shop the perimeter of the store. Most products lined up on the aisles are canned or boxed convenience foods that have been processed to oblivion in most cases so stick to the outer edges of the store in order to remove some guessing and label-reading from the equation.

Look for produce that is fresh and in season. Try not to just grab-and-go. Really stop and take a moment to examine the produce you are thinking of purchasing. You will need to employ all of your senses to help you pick a winner. Pick up the item that catches your eye and turn it over to check for brown spots and holes. The flesh should be firm but not rock hard and free of any dents or pits under the surface that may have occurred during shipping. Pay attention to the weight of the item in your hands. Especially with things like melons or oranges, heaviness can be the key to finding a juicy piece of fruit! Bring the item up and breathe it in. No, you do not have to make a spectacle of yourself by sniffing all of the produce in reach but you should detect a light sweet aroma. Strong or sour odor can suggest that what you are considering is approaching or already past its prime such as with melons and pineapple. Give squash and melons a little thump to determine ripeness and take that into consideration according to your meal plan. The produce planned for a meal toward the end of the week can afford to be a little less ripe than something you are cooking for dinner that night.

A number of the same rules for selecting fruit is applicable to vegetables, as well. The surface of the vegetable should be smooth, consistent, and evenly colored. An exception would be the squeeze test. Any give below the surface can indicate rotting and bruising. A firm texture is ideal. When evaluating leafy greens, you will want to observe a plumpness and regularity concerning the color of the leaves. You will want your greens to be smooth and snappy. However, some slight breakage and browning is a common side effect of the shipping process. If the majority of the leaves are smooth and unbroken, the few casualties of shipping can be looked over. Root vegetables such as carrots, turnips, potatoes, radishes, and onions should be firm and tough. If you notice any cracks and crevices around the base, it is an indicator that the vegetable has started to dry out.

Some produce will be shipped to stores with a wax coating in order to preserve freshness and prevent bruises during transit. Many fruits and vegetables produce a natural wax to help retain moisture which is usually washed off during processing and replaced with an artificial likeness. Keep this in mind when making your decision. An apple, for example, that is red and shiny but soft under the surface is probably not the best choice. If you buy produce that has been treated with wax, there is a method to removing it once you get home. Begin by getting rid of any stickers then gently scrub the surface under cold water a soft vegetable brush with to remove dirt and residue. Finally, plug your sink, fill it about halfway to the top with cold water, then add 3 or 4 cups of vinegar to make a solution depending on the volume of water you are using. The ideal ratio is 1 part vinegar to 3 parts water. Plunk your fruit into the solution and let it sit for about ten minutes.

A few tips for frugal folks: Shop in bulk. Some grocery chains display loose unpackaged foods such as nuts, olives, grains, and legumes. The cost that producers save on packaging is usually passed onto the consumer. Also, this way you can control the portion you buy to avoid spoiling. Bonus points for bringing reusable containers to store your goods! Avoid convenience foods. For example: vegetables that have already been chopped, bagged ready-to-eat salads, and shredded cabbage. These will more than likely cost much more than whole produce, create unnecessary waste due to the packaging, and more often than not are treated with even more preservatives to keep them fresh on the shelf for a longer period of time. Try to plan a few meals with alternative protein sources. Swapping an animal protein once a week for lentils, black beans, or tofu is going to make your wallet happy and reduce your fat intake without sacrificing on protein.

Chapter 9: Tips & Tricks To Eating Clean

Besides eating quality, naturally nutritious foods there are a few ideas that can help you reach your full potential and propel you to the next level of healthy living.

The following principles are based on nutrition science and common sense. If properly applied they can make a huge difference in your health, energy level and appearance, as I said, beside the good, clean food you eat.

Combinations

We all combine foods when we eat yet we do it based on outdated, possibly unhealthy traditions and most of us really don't even have the faintest idea what we are doing and end up combining whatever feels good to us but not necessarily what is good to our well-being.

Combining two or more types of foods may actually amplify or mute certain effects in your body. In other words, the mere simultaneous presence of certain biochemical substances in you may determine what your body will do and how it will react to them.

Certain foods do really well with others therefore exerting a powerful synergistic effect on your body. It could be what we consider good or bad. Some other food combinations only have a weak synergy together therefore their presence will not have a pronounced effect on your biochemistry.

Portions

Portion control may be one of the most crucial aspects of eating healthy! In our time and day, we generally tend to overeat. As a matter of fact, overeating seems to be a widely accepted first world problem although the acceptable portions tend to differ from one culture to another. One of the worst statistics originate from the United States which should not be a surprise; just look at the sizes of US fast food portions and the sugary drinks that come with them!

The proper portion size is different for everyone. Determining it requires to take your weight, sex, age, metabolic rate, body type, body composition and many other related factors into consideration.

Although the scope of this publication is not this, the general rule of thumb regarding a proper portion size is simple; eat only as much as will make you feel "un-hungry" but not quite full. In classic nutritionist writings, this amount measures to a not very scientific "one and a half cupped handful" of food, assuming you eat high quality, nutritious food at least 5 times a day, 2-3 hours apart.

Here is the biomechanics of overeating:

When you eat more than you should the wall of your stomach will start stretching, thus making your stomach bigger. You will want to feel the same «fullness» at your next meal so you overeat again and the same thing will happen. So the evil cycle is: filling up more room requires eating more food. Eating more food makes your stomach bigger. Now there is even more room in your stomach to be filled! So you need more food... I am sure you can see a repeating cycle emerging here. This is the general cause for most bulging guts, if not necessarily the direct cause for excess body fat.

Timing

Timing can also be responsible for a lot of good, if done right and a lot of misery, if done poorly. If you nail timing your meals then you start eating when you should and stop when you should, but it is not just when you eat but how often you eat.

If your meals are too close to each other, your metabolism may instantly pay the price; your digestion probably won't have enough time to fully process your meal before your next one, thus not being able to digest to its full potential.

If it is the other way around and your meals are too far apart, your blood sugar levels may dramatically drop so your brain won't be able to function properly, your body may go into emergency mode slowing down your metabolism wreaking havoc in your system.

The Four White Devils

Another great and simple way (also a perfect first step towards eating clean) is to avoid the Four White Devils. Sometimes these are also referred to as the Four Horsemen of Fat-O-Calypse:

- White flour
- Sugar
- Animal fats and dairy
- Salt

While there is still a vehement debate going on whether which one of these substances, if any, are actually so harmful that you need to avoid them completely, I found it advisable to consume these with a lot of caution. It is good to be aware of what they can do to you in certain quantities, if eaten on a regular basis but leaving them behind altogether is also a great option, as the lack of them will not cause any damage to your body.

Success Stories

Switching to eating clean is well known to have incredible ramifications in one's life!

I have experienced what it can do first hand, in my life, but I have also seen how it helped others even when all hope seemed to have gone.

Please read these stories and know that these aren't the only ones around but in my opinion these display the hidden healing power of eating clean robustly.

I changed the names of individuals to protect identities and preserve their privacy.

The Story of N

N has always been a naturally skinny little girl, then a skinny teenager and a skinny adult. Although being naturally skinny is what most people only dream about it isn't always a dream. N was born and raised in Eastern Europe so obviously she has been brought up with her Eastern European country's eating traditions, as for the everyday norm. Needless to say, these traditions are way outdated and nutritionally speaking disastrous. N felt it too as she had a bunch of medical conditions or better yet a rather huge collection of medical conditions that didn't disrupt her life but made it very inconvenient for her and sometimes even borderline unbearable.

These included an almost permanent migraine, a very unhealthy skin tone, huge, inflamed acnes on her back, cellulitis, extremely strong foot odor, warts on her hands, fungus on her feet, too much sweating, feminine problems (like irregular menstrual cycles, menstrual aches), hormonal problems, breast tension and super-sensitivity just to mention the worst ones.

The contrast is also interesting. A few short months after N transitioned to eating clean most of these issues seemed to have normalized and finally completely disappeared when N went all the way and minimized the animal originated foods in her diet. She ultimately became a vegetarian, the kind who still eats fish, dairy and eggs - only no meat and her recent blood tests 14 years later are actually better than ever: her red blood cell count is perfect, minerals are way above normal, her white blood cell regulation is super and all of this is with a very healthy, naturally regulated low blood pressure.

Another interesting fact about N: she was already a clean eater vegetarian when she got pregnant with her first son M. The older, traditionally eating females in her family advised her to eat meat and heavy, greasy pork/potato based foods so she can have a healthy child. N, of course, refused to give in as she already knew the beneficial effects of eating clean. Nine months later she gave birth to a very healthy, strong boy, M. While N only had gained about 4 pounds in total during her pregnancy.

A further interesting fact is that her son M has always been eating very similarly to N despite the fact that bad, traditional eating habits were constantly present around them in their family yet they didn't seem to have been much of an influence, let alone temptation, to either of them. Interestingly, M says this kind of eating clean and healthy gives him an incredible amount of comfort that he can't really explain. This shouldn't come as a surprise as we know a pregnant mother shares almost all the nutrients in her blood stream with the fetus in her womb through the placenta. Recent studies suggest that our first memories form in our mother's womb. These early memories could be anything from sounds (like the mother's heartbeat) or just being in the fetus position or even «feeling» a certain way due to the given shared chemical balance. These memories seem to stay with us for the rest of our lives embedded deeply in the foundations of our psyche. If you connect these two bits of information you may have a hypothesis on your hands: if the baby's first memories are of the «healthy-chemistry» kind and they may link to feeling safe and loved, hence he will strive for it subconsciously or otherwise through the entirety of his life.

The Story of V

V was actually related to N. She was N's sister in law and was one of the family members that teased N and gave her a really hard time when she started her transition to eating clean as a vegetarian. It is but ironic that years after being as nasty to N as one can get V was diagnosed with a very serious case of rapidly worsening sclerosis multiplex. It crippled her quickly more and more day after day.

Desperately and unsuccessfully trying a series of modern medical approaches V was about to give up. By this time her sclerosis multiplex had advanced so much she was almost 100% wheelchair bound and in an incredible amount of pain.

Acting on N's advice, almost as a last resort, V consulted with a natural healer who recommended her a new lifestyle of eating clean, and in her case, a strictly organic raw vegan diet.

Shortly after entirely switching out her eating habits V's situation gradually became better until she seemed to have fully recovered without any leftover symptoms.

Now, it is debatable whether her full recovery was due to eating clean or the actual strict organic raw vegan diet but I'd say it was the mixture of both and it being organic had the main role. You may follow a raw vegan diet but you may still want to eat as clean as possible for best results; you just can't get around eating quality foods if you want to eat clean. Either way, V's story is a true testament to what difference your diet or your eating habits can make in your life.

Almost a decade after her seemingly fatal diagnosis, V is still gladly on her raw vegan regiment free of symptoms: she studies languages, regularly takes yoga classes and as productive, mobile and happy as one can get.

The Story of C

Now, C was a real wild child. A party animal from his early teen years, trying out everything and anything that could alter his mind and didn't care if it changed his body. This included alcohol, cigarettes and drugs of all sorts. So far away from being healthy, let alone being health conscious his focus was not at all on eating cleaner. He was really heavy, weighing about 220 lbs. Also he was visibly «puffed up» and undernourished at the same time. (Technically, a big, fat guy with skinny arms.) It was not until his mid twenties when he realized that he couldn't go on living like that. The sudden, surprising death of a few of his friends gave him the initial jolt to do a thorough self review. This is when he started to clean up his act: he quit doing drugs, drinking and even smoking. All within a year. Then he started focusing on living a healthier life. This included sweating at least three times a week for at least 30 minutes, drinking more filtered water and cutting out the crap food. Later the latter one changed to eating better quality foods.

He didn't have the help of a nutritionist because he couldn't afford one. He didn't have the internet's help either because this story is taking place in a pre-internet «for-information-go-to-the-library» kind of stone age era called the early nineties. It took C about 15 years to learn and figure out the basics of healthy nutrition and realize that the more you know the more you realize how much you still don't!

He is still learning today but he is relatively more knowledgeable than most people so he actually counts as one of the leading authorities in this regard.

Yes, it is my story. I am C.

Chapter 10: Clean Eating Meal Plan

If you decide to swap out any of the recipes or whole foods in this meal plan for something else, remember that clean eating is very similar to the paleo diet. You should stick with whole, fresh foods over any processed or packaged foods, and try to keep it simple. Dieters often fail because they make things too complex, which leads to frustration and eventually giving up.

Let's get started with your clean eating, fifteen-day meal plan!

15 Day Clean Eating Meal Plan

	Breakfast	Lunch	Dinner
Sunday	Leftover Breakfast Casserole with Sausages	Orange Tempeh Stir Fry	Easy Roast Chicken
Monday	Flourless Banana Pancakes	Strawberry and Basil Salad	Chicken with Brussels Sprouts
Tuesday	Paleo Pancakes	Endive and Escarole Salad	Quinoa Salad
Wednesday	Cherry Tomato and Basil Quiche	Eggplant Mykonos	Carrot Soup with Yogurt
Thursday	Fruit Salad	Smoky Chipotle Vegetarian Bowl	Spicy Tuna Cakes
	Spaghetti Squash	Carrot and Snap	Leek and

Friday	**Breakfast Bowl**	Pea Salad	Sweet Potatoes Soup
Saturday	**Breakfast Casserole with Sausages**	Cabbage and Carrot Salad	Lime Chicken Wings

	Breakfast	Lunch	Dinner
Sunday	Chocolate Avocado Strawberry Smoothie	Orange Tempeh Stir Fry	Lime Chicken Wings
Monday	Paleo Pancakes	Eggplant Mykonos	Quinoa Salad
Tuesday	Cherry Tomato and Basil Quiche	Cabbage and Carrot Salad	Spicy Tuna Cakes
Wednesday	Fruit Salad	Strawberry and Basil Salad	Leek and Sweet Potatoes Soup
Thursday	Flourless Banana Pancakes	Carrot and Snap Pea Salad	Chicken with Brussels Sprouts
Friday	Breakfast Casserole with Sausages	Endive and Escarole Salad	Easy Roast Chicken
Saturday	Spaghetti Squash Breakfast Bowl	Smoky Chipotle Vegetarian Bowl	Carrot Soup with Yogurt

	Breakfast	Lunch	Dinner
Sunday	Pumpkin Pie Smoothie	Cabbage and Carrot Salad	Easy Roast Chicken
Monday	Fruit Salad	Endive and Escarole Salad	Lime Chicken Wings
Tuesday	Flourless Banana Pancakes	Strawberry and Basil Salad	Carrot Soup with Yogurt
Wednesday	Paleo Pancakes	Smoky Chipotle Vegetarian Bowl	Chicken with Brussels Sprouts
Thursday	Spaghetti Squash Breakfast Bowl	Eggplant Mykonos	Quinoa Salad
Friday	Cherry Tomato and Basil Quiche	Orange Tempeh Stir Fry	Leek and Sweet Potatoes Soup
Saturday	Breakfast Casserole with Sausages	Carrot and Snap Pea Salad	Spicy Tuna Cakes

Remember, you can substitute whole foods, salad, or any simple dish that doesn't involve adding too many processed foods for any of the recipes mentioned in the meal plan. Just be sure to stay away from extra sugar and processed foods with refined grains and sugars in them.

Chapter 11: Eating clean on the go

With the hectic schedules many of us keep, it's often hard to avoid falling into bad eating habits. So how do you keep up with clean eating at school, work, the soccer game? Again planning and preparation are the keys. Setting aside a block of time to prep your food for the week saves twice the time later, even if you're not eating clean! Sometimes it's as simple as making a double-batch of lasagna and freezing half for a no-fuss meal next week, or mixing up and baking two casseroles at once for an eat-one-freeze-one special. Simmer up a triple pot of chili. These types of meals can also be saved as individual portions for quick microwavable lunches or dinners. Cooking several meals at once is also nice for your utility bill!

Pre-prep and package your vegetables for snacks, lunch boxes, or quick stir-fry's later on. Make ahead and freeze your own piecrust for quick hearty quiches or potpies. Go further, make and freeze whole fruit pies in season for baking months later! I remember my mother doing this. She'd get the "seconds" from local fruit farms---the fruit that was misshapen, too small or large, or had minor blemishes on the skin. They may not be as attractive for just eating but they're perfect for cooking! Then she'd spend a day making and freezing pies. She saved a ton of money, and we enjoyed fresh baked peach or apple pies in the depths of winter.

And, definitely dust off that crock-pot! Slow cookers not only give you a hot meal without the fuss when you get home. They can help you prepare ahead of time for meals to come. Cook chicken overnight in the slow cooker, put the whole crock in the fridge in the morning, and slice or cube the chicken later. You can use it for dinner, freeze it, or both. You'll save time and money, and you'll still be able to eat clean! The same goes for soups and many other dishes. Your crock-pot can even help you with having a healthy "clean" breakfast, ready when you get up. Oatmeal is fantastic slow-cooked overnight! A slow-cooker cookbook can get you started---just substitute clean ingredients in the recipes. The possibilities are endless, and once you begin you'll quickly come up with your own.

Stock your pantry with nuts, pumpkin seeds, organic raisins, and other clean snack foods. Apart from snacking, substitute them for commercial potato chips in lunch boxes. There's a large variety of dried fruits in the organic section of the store that work very well for this, as do "clean" pretzels. Please don't forget eggs---a hard-boiled egg makes a healthy and protein-filled addition to either breakfast or lunch, and they can be prepared ahead of time and kept peeled in the refrigerator for quick packing or eating.

Fitting new eating habits into your busy lifestyle isn't hard if you take some time to plan for it. You may also find that the preparation time becomes a relaxing ritual for you. Dicing veggies or peeling apples doesn't require a lot of thought or attention, leaving your mind free to mull over other matters. The mechanical motions can also be very soothing. I know a couple who devote one Saturday morning a month to making their own "clean" bread. They've done it for years---mixing, kneading, talking, and just spending time together. They decompress from their high-pressured workweek and fill their freezer with great healthy bread at the same time! Definitely a win-win!

Chapter 12: Eating Clean for Weight Loss

If you want to shed some pounds, you'll need to follow some stricter guidelines. Eating clean won't automatically melt off the excess weight. It's not a magic bullet, no matter what some web sites may want you to believe. You'll need to focus on portion control, protein-carb balance, when you eat, and the actual nutrients in your food. Of course, adding extra physical activity helps as well!

Portion control is huge if you expect to lose weight. You know the dangers of "supersize me", but many people anymore are unaware of just what a normal size serving should be. It's been a long time since we've seen them! Even dinner plates have been supersized in the past 40 years! Standard everyday plates used to be 9 inches; it's hard nowadays to find any plates smaller than 10 ½ and many are 12 inches. That's a huge increase in surface area because it increases exponentially. An inch increase in diameter is much more than an inch more surface area. [Ask a math person and they can explain it to you.] What this means to portion control is that your normal sized serving looks inadequate and lost on your enormous plate! If you have what are called luncheon plates, usually 8 to 8½ inches, try using those. Your "normal" portions will fill your plate more pleasingly and it will look like more food. A psychological trick, yes, but it works! And you'll begin to scale back your eyes from the "supersize me" trap.

So what is a single serving? For meat and fish, it's generally the size of your palm, for veggies or starches, the size of your fist. Using this sort of "eyeball measure" helps you to see how much you're eating, even when you eat out. Most restaurants are really giving you double or triple servings. Eyeballing is also much quicker and easier than trying to weigh or measure everything. You can also picture your plate (not a jumbo plate!) as divided in 5 sections. You should have one of lean protein, one of healthy carb, and three of fruits and veggies.

Tosca Reno, who popularized clean eating, recommends that you write down your goals before you begin to help keep you focused---and keep them realistic! Starting your day with a good breakfast, such as oatmeal with fresh berries and a hard-boiled egg, will keep you feeling full all day, not just all morning. It has a long-term effect on both satiety and metabolism. Graze! Eat small amounts every 2-3 hours for optimal weight loss. This keeps your metabolism revved up, and it's a habit of naturally thin people.

To lose weight with clean eating, you also need to keep a closer watch on the nutrients in your food. Pair your proteins and carbs, and keep them in balance as much as possible. You'll need to limit your carbs to about 100-150g per day, and that's total carbs, which includes fruits and vegetables. You should also limit your intake of fruit due to its high sugar content since sugar of any kind makes you crave more sugar. But also avoid under-eating! It gives you less calories, true, but it slows your entire metabolism so you don't burn up the calories. Be aware of not just how much but also what you're eating.

We also need to return to dairy here for a minute. Apart from being processed foods, low-fat and nonfat dairy are not good for weight loss. Really. A 2005 study found that reduced-fat dairy products were actually associated with weight gain! Yikes!!! Whether this is due to the processing or to the addition of ingredients to compensate for the loss in taste, you're better off and will feel more satisfied with eating full fat dairy. I know this flies in the face of what you've been told for so long, but it appears to be true. Full fat plain yogurt with your own fruit added will help you shed pounds better than the reduced fat versions. If it's a little too tart for you, add some honey---and ditch that "healthy" spread in favor of real butter while you're at it.

Eat only until you're "contented" not "full". Eating more slowly helps you to learn to recognize when you've reached this point. Put away the rest for later; if eating out, bring the extra home. Naturally slim people do this all the time, so it's a habit that will help you not only lose weight but maintain that weight loss. "Half now, half later" is a weight control mantra that will serve you well. Learn to listen to your body.

Keeping your water intake levels high is also very important for weight loss. You should consume at least 2-3 liters a day. We need water more than food. I'm sure you've heard that three days without water will kill you, but it takes three weeks to starve! Dehydration is often mistaken for hunger, so adequate water is necessary to help keep your diet on track. It also assists in flushing toxins from your system on a regular basis. The first couple of days you'll need to visit the restroom more often, it's true, but your body will soon accept that it's finally getting adequate water and it'll adjust.

You'll also need to limit your caffeine intake since it's a natural diuretic causing you to lose water. This is a hard one for many people! If you're eating clean, you've already cut out the myriad soft drinks, energy drinks, and "health" drinks that contain caffeine because of their other ingredients. Try substituting some green or herbal teas (hot or chilled), or some lemonade made with a low calorie natural sweetener like honey or stevia. Don't, however, substitute them for your water. It's water, then other beverages!

It's also important to be aware of some items know as "diet-busters", healthy foods that can undo your weight loss plan and progress if you're not very careful with them. The first is granola, even clean homemade granola. It's very dense, and a serving size is actually very small, making it easy to eat too much. It's also heavily carb-laden and can increase your appetite for the entire day, so be wary. The next potential diet-buster is hummus. It's very popular right now, and, yes, it's very healthy. Hummus is also high fat so portions need to be very small. Again it's an easy item to overeat. Peanut butter...ditto.

The final two diet-busters have become ubiquitous, and, like the previous ones, they're sneaky. The first of them is smoothies. The readily available versions you'll find at the mall (or even health clubs) are usually supersized, giving you several servings in one container. They also often contain added sugar through using sugared fruit to improve the taste. This is a tricky weight-loss trap---"I only had a smoothie!" You may actually have downed three or four servings, along with many times your daily allotment of carbs! The same type of thing is true for diet-buster number five, wraps. The wrapper itself is dense and often large. Many are equivalent to three slices of bread! Their size also disguises just how much filling is rolled up in there. It can often be far more than a normal sandwich! To keep both of these items from deep-sixing your weight loss efforts, make your own. If you're buying them when you're out and about, greatly reduce the portion size by sharing with a friend or saving some for later. As with most of the diet-busters, the food itself is good for you but portion control is vital!

A final caveat for achieving your weight loss goals: avoid "diet" products. Very few protein bars, for instance, are clean and most contain quite a bit of sugar. They may have a good protein-carb balance but they're not using healthy carbs to do it. The same goes for diet shakes or drinks. You'll do better, feel more satisfied, and lose more weight if you stick with real food in controlled portions. After all, that's what clean eating is really all about, isn't it?

Chapter 13: Common Clean Eating Mistakes

1. Still Overeating

People who try to eat clean sometimes forget the importance of being mindful of how much they eat. Some feel that since what they are eating is considered healthy and organic, they could eat as much as they want. Keeping track of your calorie intake is not necessary when you are clean eating. However, you still need to consider the fact that how much you eat is just as important as what you eat. To avoid this mistake, you need to determine your required daily caloric intake and not go above that. Remember that for you to achieve a healthier lifestyle, you still need to downsize portions and control the amount of food that you eat.

2. Shopping on an empty stomach

If there's one thing that you should not do while grocery shopping is doing it on an empty stomach. When you decide to go on shopping even if you're hungry, you are more likely to choose and buy food without even thinking about them. According to experts, if you shop on an empty stomach, you are more likely to grab high-calorie foods. So, when you decide to go on grocery shopping, eat a snack before entering the store. It would also help if you have prepared a grocery-shopping list to make sure that you'll by everything you need and not go beyond your budget.

3. Not making homemade meals

Whole foods are best prepared at home. This is because you are fully in control of how you handle and spice up your meal. By learning how to prepare and cook your own meals you can eat what you want and when you want to eat them. You no longer have to settle for take-outs or microwaveable meals. Try your best to prepare meal plans during the weekends so that no matter how busy you are from Mondays to Fridays, you already have something in mind to prepare and eat when you get home.

4. Not Properly Spacing Out Your Meals

Another common mistake of people who go on a clean eating diet is that they forget to properly time or space out their meals. Experts suggests that its best to have at least 6 mini meals a day spaced 2.5-3 hours apart. Remember that skipping a meal will not help you in losing weight. It would only cause you to eat more on your next meal. Planning your meals and proper timing is key if you want to successfully lose or maintain weight through clean eating.

5. Eating the same meal over and over

A lot of people who engage in clean eating often fall into a food rut. Because of their busy schedules, they tend to have staples for breakfast, lunch, dinner and snacks. Eating the same meals over and over is not only unexciting, but it also causes you to lack on the nutrients that you need.

The great thing about clean eating is that you are not restricted to eating one kind of dish over and over. You are free to experiment and learn new recipes as long as they are healthy and delicious. There are a lot of great, clean recipes that you could try. In time, you'll completely forget about all the processed and junk food because you'll love and enjoy all the healthy recipes that clean eating offers.

6. Having frequent cheat days

If you still want to have a cheat day, you should only have it once a week, at most. It feels great to chomp on a whole bag of chips or a pint of ice cream whenever you successfully go through a rather stressful day at work. However, indulging on too many cheat meals would not help with your transition to a clean eating lifestyle. Fortunately, the solution to this problem is simple. Instead of rewarding yourself with comfort food, think of other non-food rewards. This could be a day at the spa, a visit at your favorite spot or a new pair of shoes.

As you have read in the previous chapters, clean eating is a very simple and easy way to achieve a healthier and better lifestyle. There are only a few basic principles that you need to follow in order to successfully practice and develop a new way of life. When you become mindful of these common mistakes, you will be less prone to committing them. If you are guilty of doing at least one of the aforementioned examples, do not be too hard on yourself. Don't let these little mistakes hinder you from improving your health and body with clean eating strategies.

Chapter 14: Energy-Boosting Breakfast Recipes

Let's face it. It's really hard for almost everyone to wake up early in the morning to prepare food for breakfast, resulting for a drive-thru in fast food restaurants or simply missing the most important meal of the day. However, skipping breakfast can be very harmful to your clean eating lifestyle. Why would that be possible when I haven't even added a calorie on my body?

But tell you what, this often leads to excessive eating of snacks or disproportionate meals during lunch and dinner. I know, there's one more thing that drives you nuts, and that is thinking, eating healthy means being stuck on tasteless menus. Well, worry no more, the breakfast recipes in this chapter are surely delectable, satisfying, will give you a surge of energy, and more importantly, are healthy; most of them are easy to make too!

Tortilla with eggs and beans

Ingredients
- 1 scallion, sliced
- 3 teaspoons canola oil divided
- ¼ teaspoon salt divided
- 1 (15-ounce) can of pinto beans, rinsed
- 8 (6-inch) corn tortillas
- ¾ cup of shredded sharp Cheddar cheese
- 1 ½ cups of romaine lettuce, very thinly sliced
- 2 tablespoons of chopped fresh cilantro
- ½ cup of prepared green salsa

- Canola oil cooking spray
- 2 teaspoons of lime juice
- 4 large eggs
- ¼ teaspoon of pepper, freshly ground & divided

Procedure

Preheat oven to 400 degrees F. Mix 1/8 teaspoon of pepper, 1/8 teaspoon of salt, lime juice, 1 teaspoon of oil, cilantro, scallion, and lettuce in a bowl, and set aside. Combine salsa and beans in a separate bowl.

Brush the cooking spray on either side of the tortillas, and place them on a large baking sheet in four sets of overlying pairs. Scoop approximately one-third cup of the bean mix and spread over the tortillas. Sprinkle each with three tablespoons of cheese.

In the meantime, add the two teaspoons of oil left in a large nonstick skillet over medium heat. Beat the eggs in a small bowl, and then add them to the pan. Season with the remaining salt and pepper.

Lower the heat and cook for five to seven minutes while undisturbed until set.

Assemble by placing an egg over each tortilla pair, and top with a quarter cup of the lettuce mix.

Servings: 4

Breakfast taco

Ingredients

- 1 tablespoon of salsa
- ½ cup of liquid egg substitute
- 2 corn tortillas
- 2 tablespoons of shredded reduced-fat Cheddar cheese

Procedure

Top the tortillas with cheese and salsa. Slide into the microwave and heat for about thirty seconds or until the cheese has melted.

In the meantime, spread cooking spray around a small nonstick skillet, and heat over medium-high heat. Stir in your egg substitute, and cook while stirring until cooked through, approximately ninety seconds. Split the scrambled eggs among the tacos.

Serves: 2

Egg in Marinara Dressing

Gear up for this exciting meal packed with protein and essential nutrients.

Ingredients

2 fresh eggs

1/2 finely sliced onion

crushed red pepper

1 cup marinara sauce

2 whole wheat pita pocket

Procedure

1. Lightly toast the pita pocket in an oven toaster. Set aside.

Pour in olive oil in a small frying pan over medium heat.
2. Sauté onion until golden or brown.
3. Season with pepper and add the marinara sauce. Crack the eggs onto the mixture, then let it simmer.

Serve with pita pockets.

Serves: 2

Calories: 306 per serving

Baked Mushroom with Baby Spinach

Eating mushrooms can help you prevent breast cancer, high cholesterol levels, and prostate cancer. Spinach on the other hand, is loaded with protein, fiber, and vitamins A, C, E, and B6. Try this mushroom-spinach combo recipe for a nutritious breakfast!

Ingredients

2 slices of whole-wheat bread, toasted

1 cup mushrooms, cut into slices

4 tbsp. onion, chopped

3 tbsp. red bell pepper, sliced

2 cups baby spinach

4 organic eggs

salt and black pepper to taste

Procedure

1. Preheat oven to 450°F.

Coat a large pan with cooking spray. Sauté the mushrooms, onion, and bell pepper, and baby spinach for about 5 minutes.

2. Stir 4 eggs with ½ cup skim milk.
3. Pour over toasted bread then top with sautéed vegetables. Add desired amount of Parmesan cheese.

Bake for about 15 minutes.

4. Serve.

Serves: 2

Calories: 290 per serving

Cinnamon and Oats Bowl

Break every bleak weather and warm your tummy with this tasty treat.

Ingredients

2 tsp. cinnamon, freshly ground

8 tsp. brown sugar

3 cups rolled oats, organic

½ cup raisins

½ cup walnuts, chopped

low-fat milk (optional)

Procedure

1. Prepare your organic oats according to package directions.

In a mixing bowl, combine brown sugar and cinnamon. Pour over the oats.

2. Add walnuts and raisins. Stir well.
3. Splash milk if desired.

Serves: 10

Calories: 327 per 1 cup serving

Coco-Quinoa Burgoo with Strawberry

Bored with the usual oats for breakfast? Try this porridge topped with shredded coconut and strawberries.

Ingredients

6 tbsp. coconut oil

1 tsp. cinnamon, finely ground

½ cup quinoa, well rinsed

½ cup light coconut milk (preferably organic)

½ cup low-fat milk

2 tsp. maple syrup

3 tsp. shredded coconut, unsweetened

½ cup strawberries, freshly sliced

Procedure

1. Over medium heat, drizzle oil in a saucepan.

2. Add cinnamon, then quinoa and stir persistently until smoothly covered.

3. Spill both coconut and low-fat milk in the pan. Bring to a simmer until milk has been fully blended in the mixture.

4. Drizzle with maple syrup and then transfer into a bowl. Top with shredded coco and strawberries.

Serves: 2

Calories: 150 per serving

Chia Soleil Pudding

Did you know that chia seeds contain more Omega 3-s than a regular salmon? Surprised? Well, this magical seed has more to offer!

Ingredients

1 ½ cups almond milk

4 tbsp. chia seeds

1 tsp. maple syrup

½ cup fresh blueberries

For toppings:

1 ripe mango, freshly sliced

6 fresh blueberries

Procedure

1. Whip all the ingredients together in a large bowl except the toppings.

Cover and chill in the fridge for about 3 hours.

2. Remove and add up the toppings.
3. Serve and enjoy every spoonful of it!

Serves: 2

Calories: 110 per serving

Kiwi and Banana Super Bowl

Power-up each morning with this super bowl, loaded with dietary fiber that aids digestion and enhances weight loss.

Ingredients

½ cup almond milk, unsweetened

4 tbsp. ripe mango, frozen

4 tbsp. avocado, cut into cubes for easy blending

½ cup kale

½ cup spinach

3 ice cubes

¼ cup water (add more if preferred)

For the toppings:

1 regular banana, chopped

1 medium size sliced kiwi

1 tbsp. coco flakes

Procedure

1. In a clean blender, mix all the smoothie ingredients until evenly blended.

Pour in a medium sized bowl and top with banana, kiwi, and coconut flakes.

2. Serve and dig in this irresistible smoothie.

Serves: 1

Calories: 170 per serving

Creamy Salmon-Capers

Need a speedy savory satisfaction for your hectic morning schedule? You've got the perfect meal on this one.

Ingredients

½ cup cream cheese

100 g flaked salmon (cooked or canned)

1 tbsp. capers, well drained

1 tsp. lemon zest

1 whole-grain pita

1 tomato, thinly sliced into four

1 cup fresh arugula leaves

¼ cup water (add more if preferred)

Procedure

1. Combine cheese and capers in a small bowl.

Add the lemon zest. Stir well.

2. Spread the mixture half of the pita, then top with salmon flakes, tomato and arugula.
3. Fold and slice into two.

Best served with Chia Soleil Pudding.

Serves: 2

Calories: 105 per serving

Nutty Cookies with a Twist

Bored with the usual cookies with nuts? Try this recipe with added banana for a good source of omega-3 fatty acids, Vitamin E, and B Vitamins.

Ingredients

½ cup oats

1 egg, beaten

6 tbsp. low-fat milk

1 medium-sized banana, mashed

1tbsp. raisins

1 tbsp. flaxseed, finely ground

1tbsp. walnuts, chopped

1 tsp. honey

1tsp cinnamon

salt to taste

Procedure

1. Preheat the oven to 350 °F.

Place the oats in a blender until powdered.

2. In a large bowl, whisk all the ingredients together.
3. Coat a baking sheet with non-stick spray.

Scoop a batter on the sheet.

4. Bake for about 15 minutes. Serve.

Serves: 2

Calories: 150 per serving

Slow-cooked Sorghum in Pumpkin Purée

Prepare in the evening and get ready to wake-up for a bowl of whole-grain with high levels of antioxidant.

Ingredients

2 cups sorghum, thoroughly rinsed

2 cups almond milk

2 cups water

1 ½ cups pumpkin purée

2 tbsp. pumpkin pie, spiced

2 tsp. vanilla extract

Procedure

1. Combine all ingredients in a slow cooker. Stir well and let it simmer over low fire for 8 hours.
2. Serve.

Serves: 8

Calories: 221 per serving

Rainbow Acai in a Jar

Enjoy a breakfast filled with colorful fruits on jars that even kids will surely love!

Ingredients

2 packs acai purée, frozen

1 regular banana

1 mango, finely sliced

1 kiwi, cubed

2 tbsp. nuts, unsalted and chopped

1 cup fresh raspberries

1tbsp. coconut, unsweetened and shredded

4tbsp coconut milk

¼ cup water

Procedure

1. In a food processor or blender, combine acai, milk, and water. Blend well until you achieve a smooth consistency.

Pour in the mixture evenly on jars then layer fruits, nuts and coconut.

2. Cover and freeze to fridge.

Serves: 2

Calories: 296 per serving

Chapter 15: Spice-up Every Lunch with Healthy Fully-loaded Meals

Not sure what to eat during lunch time? You don't have to stick with the usual salad in the office. Satisfy and fill your stomach with these delectable meals that's below 500 calories.

Chile-crusted scallops with cucumber salad

Ingredients

Salad

- ½ cup of cashews salted roasted & coarsely chopped
- 2 teaspoons of lemon juice
- ¼ cup of coarsely chopped flat-leaf parsley
- 2 medium cucumbers
- 2 thinly sliced scallions, (white & light green parts)
- ¼ cup of extra-virgin olive oil
- 1/8 teaspoon of salt

Scallops

- 2 tablespoons of minced seeded serrano chile
- ½ teaspoon of kosher salt
- 1 teaspoon of cumin seeds
- 1 teaspoon of freshly cracked black pepper
- ¼ pounds of dry sea scallops

Procedure

For the salad: peel the cucumbers, and seed them. Divide them lengthwise and slice into quarter inch thick pieces. Combine the parsley, oil, lemon juice, scallions, cashews, cucumbers and salt in a large bowl.

For the scallops: Toss the cumin seeds into a small skillet and toast them over medium high heat or until fragrant, approximately one minute. Place on a cutting board and allow to cool before chopping coarsely. Combine the salt, pepper, chile, and cumin seeds in a small bowl. Drain the scallops, then pat and rub using the spice mixture. Thread scallops on 4-quarter inch skewers.

Warm your grill to medium high, and spray the grill rack with oil. Grill scallops for approximately four minutes per side. Remove scallops carefully and serve warm with cucumber salad.

Servings: 4

Hearty Ham Sandwich

The whole family will flip for this yummy and hearty meal, loaded with cheesy ham.

Ingredients

1tsp. butter

4 mushrooms, thinly sliced

4 slices whole-wheat bread

4 slices Swiss cheese

4 slices roasted ham, uncured

Procedure

1. Preheat a panini press.

Melt butter in a skillet over medium heat.

2. Sauté mushrooms until golden. Set aside.
3. Layer the remaining ingredients between bread slices.

Place the ham sandwich in a panini press until well toasted.

4. Serve.

Serves: 4

Calories: 280 per serving

Green Leafy Wraps

Be amazed with this meat-tasting wraps that's actually made with pure veggies. Don't believe me? Taste it for yourself!

Ingredients

1tsp. butter

4 cups walnuts, coarsely ground

2 tbsp. cumin, finely ground

3 tsp. chili powder

3 tsp. coriander powder

4 tbsp. tamari

12 large collard leaves

salsa (homemade or from grocery stores)

Procedure

1. Combine all ingredients (except leaves) in a large bowl.

Spoon a mixture in the middle portion of the leaf, then top with salsa.

2. Roll the leaf ala burrito.
3. Repeat step with the remaining filling and leaves. Serve.

Serves: 12

Calories: 275 per serving

Potato Pizza

Who says you can't have pizza when on a diet? Munch this mouthwatering cheesy crust up until the last bite!

Ingredients

6 medium-sized sweet potatoes, mashed

2 cups almond flour

1 cup pizza sauce

1 cup cheese (preferably mozzarella)

2 tsp. baking soda

2 tbsp. Italian seasoning

1 tsp. salt

toppings of your choice (ham, tomatoes, bacon)

Procedure
1. Set oven to 450 °F.

In a serving bowl, mix in potatoes, baking soda, flour, seasoning, and salt.

2. Mold using your hands, until mixture forms a pizza dough.
3. Line a parchment paper in a pizza pan.

Bake for about 20 minutes.

4. Slice up and enjoy!

Serves: 4

Calories: 351 per serving

A Taste of the Caribbean

Eat up with a dish that's bursting with flavors of lime and different spices.

Ingredients

1 tuna steak, cooked and sliced into pieces

½ cup vegetable broth

½ cup mango, diced

½ red bell pepper, chopped

4 tbsp. scallions, finely cut

2 tbsp. cilantro

3 tsp. peanut butter

1 ½ tsp. rice wine vinegar

1 ½ tsp. lime juice, freshly squeezed

2 butterhead lettuce

½ cup vegetable broth

Procedure

1. Toss tuna, scallions, cilantro, and mango in a bowl. Set aside.

In another container, combine wet ingredients. Add to tuna mixture.

2. Add salt and pepper to add flavor.
3. Arrange lettuce leaves on a large plate, then put the mixture in each.

Serves: 2

Calories: 260 per serving

Shrimp in Collards

You can't resist eating this shrimp recipe for lunch after a busy morning.

Ingredients

1 kl. shrimp, peeled and deveined (remove tail if preferred)

½ kl. fresh collard greens, finely chopped

4 medium-sized shallots or any onions, thinly sliced

4 turkey sausages

4 tbsp. scallions, finely cut

2 tbsp. olive oil (divide into two)

1 tsp. spice mixture or herbs

½ tsp. sea salt

1 tsp. paprika

1 tsp. chili powder

ground black and cayenne pepper to taste

Procedure

1. Toss last five ingredients in a small bowl.

In a separate container, mix shrimp with herbs.

2. Prepare a medium wok, and put over medium-high fire.
3. Heat 1 tbsp. olive oil. Stir onions, shrimp, until turns pink in color. Set aside.

Cook sausage in the remaining oil until golden. Layer collard greens in the pan then cover for about 2 minutes.

4. Add the shrimp mixture and cook for 1 more minute.
5. Serve while hot.

Serves: 8

Calories: 268 per serving

Fruity Detox Drink

Sweet and creamy detox drink? Why not? Feel good inside and out!

Ingredients

1 cup raspberries

2 bananas, diced

1 kiwi, cut into slices

2 fresh oranges

1 cup ripe mango, frozen and chopped

¾ cup Acai purée

1 cup coco milk, unsweetened

2 fresh mint leaves

2 scoops vanilla pea, powdered

Procedure
1. Place all listed ingredients in a clean blender or a food processor.

Blend until you achieve a smooth consistency.

2. Pour into a mason jar or glass. Serve immediately.

Serves: 2

Calories: 342 per serving

Savory Steak with Salsa

Heat your taste buds with this must-try dish –a signature classic steak recipe paired with salsa.

Ingredients

olive oil cooking spray

2 tbsp. olive oil

½ kilo tenderloin steak, well washed

6 tomatoes, cut into half

6 tbsp. freshly squeezed lemon juice

2 minced garlic

1 cup cilantro leaves, chopped

black pepper, freshly ground

salt to taste

1 summer squash, cut lengthwise making 4 slices

1 fresh zucchini, slice into four

2 onions, slice into two

2 jalapeño pepper, seed removed and cut in half

Procedure

1. Preheat oven to 475 °F.

Prepare 2 large roasting pans and coat with cooking spray.

2. Arrange tomatoes and last four ingredients on the pans.
3. Place in the oven and roast for about 12 minutes.

For the dressing, put in lime juice, and garlic, salt and pepper, and cilantro in a small mixing bowl. Set aside.

4. Remove veggies from oven and let it cool for a while.
5. Cut vegetables into cubes and carefully combine them with the dressing in another container.

Pour dressing over chopped salsa and chill in the fridge.

Over medium fire, heat olive oil in a non-stick pan. Season the steak (both sides) with salt and pepper and cook in the pan for about 4 minutes on each side.

6. Serve on a large plate with a cup of veggie salsa on the side.

Serves: 8

Calories: 204 per serving

Asian-style Broccoli Noodles

Yin and yang, a famous concept of Asian cuisine which represents a perfect balance. This Asian inspired recipe has that for you— the perfect balance of flavors in a noodle dish.

Ingredients

1 tsp. olive oil

2 cups whole-wheat spaghetti noodles

10 crowns, broccoli florets

2 oranges, freshly squeezed and zested

2 cups snow peas, trimmed

4 tbsp. soy sauce

½ tsp. red pepper flakes

8 cloves minced garlic

2 tbsp. ginger, grounded

Procedure
1. In a large pot, boil water and put noodles. Stir occasionally. Add broccoli and simmer for about five minutes.
2. Remove from water and transfer to a bowl. Set aside.
3. Place orange zest and juice, soy sauce, ginger and pepper flakes in a small bowl. Whisk thoroughly.

Heat a large non-stick skillet over medium heat. Cook beef, then add peas and the mixture from the small bowl.

4. Pour in beef mixture to spaghetti and toss carefully, until well coated.

Serves: 8

Calories: 379 per serving

Tasty Turkey Tacos

This is the perfect whole-grain meal to keep your tummy full and happy.

Ingredients

6 corn tortillas

½ kilo ground lean turkey

1 cup black beans

1 bundle romaine lettuce

½ cup salsa

olive oil cooking spray

ground black pepper and salt to taste

Procedure

1. Preheat oven to 350°F.

Wrap tortillas in foil, to make 2 packets.

2. Place on a baking sheet and bake for about 15 minutes.
3. Over medium fire, coat a non-stick pan with cooking spray.

Season turkey with salt and pepper, then cook until browned.

4. Remove foil from packets and lay to plates.
5. Distribute lettuce, turkey, beans, and salsa evenly on corn tortillas.

Fold or create a wrap and serve warm.

Serves: 3

Calories: 276 per serving

Crabby-Avocado Salad

A protein-packed dish paired with avocado, providing a great creamy texture on every bite.

Ingredients

4 regular-sized avocado, sliced
½ kilo lump crabmeat, cooked
8 hard boiled eggs, cut into slices
4 tomatoes, chopped
4 shredded butter leaf lettuce
1 cup black beans
1 thinly sliced fennel bulb
2 carrots, finely chopped

For the dressing:

1 cup buttermilk
2 cups Greek yogurt (nonfat)
½ cup chili sauce
4 tbsp. onion, grated
1 clove minced garlic
1 tsp. cayenne pepper, grounded
4 tbsp. fresh parsley, finely chopped
½ tsp. salt

Procedure

1. In a medium-sized bowl, mix all the ingredients for the dressing and set aside.

On a large plate, lay lettuce (or your choice of individual serving) and top with tomatoes, eggs, carrot, fennel, crab, and avocado.

2. Serve with dressing.

Serves: 8
Calories: 246 per serving

Chapter 16: Clean Eating Dinner Recipes under 300 Cal

Mac n' Cheese Overload

Macaroni and cheese? We all know the winning pair!

Ingredients

1 ½ cup elbow macaroni (whole-grain)

1 ½ oz. roasted ham, finely diced

1 oz. mushrooms (preferable cremini), finely sliced

1 ½ tsp. brown-rice flour

1 cups low-fat milk (divide into two half cups)

1 cup Swiss cheese, grated

1/2 tbsp. mustard

1 tsp. olive oil

1 tsp. butter, unsalted

1 small onion, sliced

sea salt and black pepper to taste

herbs of your choice for garnishing

Procedure

1. Cook macaroni according to packaging instructions. Heat oil in a large pan on medium-high.
2. Sauté onion and ham until browned, then add the mushroom.
3. Sprinkle with flour, and season with salt, and pepper.

Add mustard and ½ cup milk. Stir well.
4. Gradually add the remaining ½ cup milk, and stir constantly until sauce is thickened.
5. Remove from heat and mix in cheese macaroni.

Serve with your fave herb.

Serves: 3

Calories: 299 per serving

Lamb Côtelette with Pear Sauce

Taste a dish that may have come from a high-end restaurant with this lamb loin recipe.

Ingredients

8 medium-sized lamb loin chops (trim fat)

1 ripe pear, peeled and cut into slices

½ cup apple juice

3 tsp. balsamic vinegar

½ cup beef broth

1 ½ tsp. rosemary and thyme, finely chopped

½ tsp. salt

½ tsp. ground black pepper

Procedure

1. Generously season the lamb with salt and pepper.

Heat a large skillet over medium-high heat, and cook lamb until golden. Set aside.

2. Remove any fat from skillet, and return to cooking over medium heat. Add pear, apple juice, balsamic, and broth and let it simmer for about 3 minutes.

3. Remove from heat and mix in the herbs rosemary and thyme.

Top the well-cooked lamb with pear sauce, and serve.

Serves: 4

Calories: 230 per serving

Orange Roast Salmon with Rosemary and Thyme

The classic ingredient combination of rosemary and thyme allow the palatable flavor of the salmon to shine through.

Ingredients

cooking spray

4 shallots, discard outer layer

9 radishes, cut into two

1 ½ cups salmon fillets, deboned

1 ½ tsp. olive oil

2 tsp. basil, chopped (fresh mint as alternative)

1 tsp. rosemary and thyme, finely chopped

1 fresh orange, thinly sliced

½ tsp. salt

½ tsp. ground black pepper

Procedure

1. Set the oven to 425°F.

Cover a large baking sheet with foil and coat with cooking spray.

2. Lightly place shallots and radishes. Then drizzle with oil.
3. Sprinkle with salt and pepper to taste.

Carefully toss and spread within the one layer.
4. Add the chopped rosemary and thyme and roast for about 15 minutes.
5. Press the veggies to edges of baking sheet and place the salmon in the middle part. Use the sliced orange to cover each fillet.

Return in the oven and continue roasting for about 20 minutes.

Remove the salmon from the oven, discarding the orange slices.

6. Toss with the freshly squeezed orange juice. Serve.

Serves: 2

Calories: 244 per serving

Seven Veggies with White Fish

Give this fish and veggie recipe a try; it will surely be a hit!

Ingredients

2 large potatoes, diced

2 regular-sized turnips, sliced

2 large carrots, cut into cubes

1 large zucchini, diced

1 red bell pepper, well chunked

1 cup green beans, cut into two

½ fresh green cabbage, sliced into about an inch size

1 kl. tilapia (or any whitefish), chunked

1 cup fresh cilantro, finely chopped

1 ½ cups chickpeas, canned and well drained

½ cup raisins

3 cloves minced garlic

1 tsp. chili paste

2 tbsp. spice mix

2 tbsp. olive oil

1 tsp. salt

Procedure

1. Heat olive oil in a large stew over medium fire.

Sauté garlic with spice mix until golden brown.

2. Add the first five ingredients in the pot and pour in water to fully cover veggies. Simmer for about 30 minutes.
3. Add in salt, beans, pepper, and chili paste and cook for another 15 minutes.

When cooked, cool it for about 10 minutes.

4. Pour the vegetable mixture in a blender or food processor until a soft-paste consistency is achieved.
5. Bring the mixture back on stew.

Add raisins, chickpeas, and fish. Cook and cover until fish meat flakes smoothly on fork. The fish will now steam on top of the veggie mixture.

Serve in your favorite bowl and sprinkle with chopped cilantro.

Serves: 12

Calories: 210 per serving

Chicken Dill 'N Dunk Marina

Transform this famous finger food into a gourmet dinner everyone will crave for.

Ingredients

¼ kilo chicken breast tenders, cut into strips

1 large organic egg

6 tbsp. bread crumbs

1 ½ tbsp. olive oil, divide into two

¼ cup carrot, peeled and grated

¼ cup white mushrooms, finely chopped

1 clove minced garlic

1 small onion, chopped

½ cup zucchini, grated

¼ cup tomatoes, crushed

2 tbsp. flour (whole-wheat)

1 tbsp. fresh dill, chopped

½ tsp. oregano, dried

ground black pepper and salt to taste

Procedure

1. Preheat oven to 375°F.

While waiting for the oven to set, heat the olive oil on a non-stick skillet over medium fire. Add onions and sauté until golden.

2. Add the carrots and mushrooms cook for about 5 minutes.
3. Add garlic, zucchini, and pepper. Then tomatoes and oregano. Stir occasionally until veggies are softened.

Remove from the pan and transfer to a blender. Mix until you achieved your preferred consistency for the dip. Set aside.

4. Place the mixture of pepper, and salt on a large plate and then bread crumbs and dill on the other plate.
5. Take a large bowl and whisk together the egg and with 2-3 tbsp. of water.

Now it's time for the dry-wet-dry technique. Roll 1 chicken on the flour mixture, then to the egg mixture, and dredge over breadcrumbs and place on a baking sheet lined with parchment paper. Continue the process with the remaining chicken tenders.

Heat oil in large skillet over medium-high fire. Cook each side of the chicken until golden. Repeat with all chicken tenders.

6. Bake the fried chicken in the oven for another 5 minutes.
7. Serve with the homemade sauce

Serves: 9

Calories: 107 per serving

Irish Ragoût

Control your diabetes and have stronger bones with this Irish Ragoût or stew.

Ingredients

½ kilo lamb, boneless and cut into pieces

2 cups beef broth

½ kilo Burbank potatoes, cut into slices

¼ kilo carrots, sliced

¼ cup parsnips, sliced

¾ cups fresh peas

¼ cup onions, finely chopped

1tbsp. fresh parsley leaves, finely chopped

½ tsp. ground black pepper

½ tsp. salt to taste

Procedure

1. Set oven at 250°F.

Boil lamb with onions, potatoes, carrots, and parsnips in a large pot.

2. Sprinkle with salt and pepper. Let it simmer then transfer to the oven.
3. Bake for about 2 hours, until the rich scent fill the kitchen.

Let the stew cool down for a few minutes and serve with parsley on top.

Serves: 5
Calories: 273 per serving

Aloha Skewers

Enjoy these fruity and meaty skewers for your meals.

Ingredients
1/4 kilo fresh pineapple, cut into cubes
½ kilo chicken breast, cubed
6 cherry tomatoes, rinsed and sliced
½ tbsp rice wine vinegar
1 onion, chopped
1 1/2 tsp. honey, raw
1 regular ginger, grated and divided
½ tbsp soy sauce
For the sauce:
½ kilo fresh pineapple, cubed
1 lime, zested and freshly squeezed
1 lemon, zested and squeezed
½ tbsp. honey
½ tsp. grated ginger

Procedure

1. Preheat an indoor grill.

Whisk together last four ingredients in a large bowl. Add chicken breast then cover.

2. Marinate in the fridge for about an hour.
3. For the sauce, place all ingredients into a food processor, until smoothly blended. Set aside.

Remove the marinated chicken from the refrigerator and drain.

4. Alternate chicken breast with cubed pineapples, dividing evenly on 6 skewers.
5. Grill until the chicken is cooked through

Serve.

Serves: 6

Calories: 80 per serving

Butterflied grilled chicken with chile-lime rub

Ingredients
- 2 tablespoons of extra-virgin olive oil
- 3 tablespoons of lime juice
- 1 teaspoon of ground coriander
- 1 teaspoon of dried oregano, preferably Mexican
- 1 teaspoon of freshly ground pepper
- 1 chicken
- 3 tablespoons of chile powder
- 2 teaspoons of freshly grated lime zest
- 1 tablespoon of minced garlic
- 1 teaspoon of ground cumin
- 1 ½ teaspoons of kosher salt
- Pinch of ground cinnamon

Procedure

Combine paprika or chile powder, oil, cinnamon, pepper, salt, oregano, cumin, coriander, garlic, lime zest and juice in a small bowl to create a wet paste.

Cut the chicken with kitchen shears on one side of its backbone, across the ribs. Cut the opposite side similarly and remove the backbone. Discard or save it for your stock. Place down with the cut side facing down and flatten using the heel of your hand. Smear a generous amount of the spice rub around the skin and the interior of the chicken.

Slide into a microwave friendly baking dish. Cover using plastic wrap and place in the refrigerator to stay overnight or for twenty-four hours.

Preheat grill to medium-high heat halfway, and leave the other side unheated.

Let the spice rub stay on the chicken, and place it on the grill with the skin side facing down until it starts coloring and forms char marks, approximately five minutes. Turn over then grill for five more minutes. Transfer to the unheated side of the grill and close the lid. Cook for thirty to forty minutes. Place onto a platter, allow to cool for five minutes, and then serve.

Servings: 6

Chapter 17: Bonus Smoothies and Dessert Recipes

Choco cinnamon pudding

Ingredients
- 2 tablespoons of sugar
- 1 teaspoon of cinnamon
- 2 ½ cups of fat-free milk
- ¼ cup of cornstarch
- 3 tablespoons of unsweetened cocoa
- 1 ounce of dark chocolate, sliced into small pieces

Procedure

Put all the ingredients in a saucepan, except the milk and heat over medium heat. Gradually stir in the milk, stirring constantly. Bring the mixture to a boil, and then boil again for one minute. Continue stirring.

Remove from heat and place in the fridge to cool before eating.

Servings: 4

Coconut cranberry cookies

Yields: 40 cookies

Ingredients
- 1 teaspoon of baking soda
- ½ cup of fat-free vanilla yogurt
- 1 tablespoon of ground flaxseed

- 1 cup of dried cranberries
- 2 cups of whole-wheat flour
- ½ cup of vegetable oil
- 1 ½ cup of agave syrup
- 1 cup of sweetened shredded coconut

Procedure

Preheat oven to 350 degrees F. Spread a thin layer of coconut on a cookie sheet, and toast in the preheated oven for ten minutes. Raise the temperature to 375 degrees F.

Mix the baking soda and flours and whisk together. Mix the syrup, yogurt, and oil using an electric mixer until fluffy. Stir in the flaxseed, and then fold in the toasted cranberries and coconut.

Scoop a tablespoon of the mixture onto a clean cookie sheet, and bake for eight to ten minutes.

Servings: 40 cookies

Hazelnut-Choco Balls

Don't be afraid for a choco dessert when on your clean eating diet. This no-cook recipe is less than 200 calories which you can store in fridge so you can just grab it when you crave for it.

Ingredients

2 cups hazelnut flour

1 cup hazelnuts, finely chopped

6 tbsp. dark chocolate, unsweetened

1 cup sour cherries, dried

1 ½ cups honey

1/2 cup coconut flour

2 tbsp. chia seeds (flaxseed if preferred)

1 tsp. vanilla extract

3 tsp. sesame seeds

1 cup rolled oats, old-fashioned

Procedure

1. In a blender, combine all ingredients except for oats. After a few seconds, add oats and blend for one more minute.

Put mixture in a large mixing bowl.

2. Wrap in plastic foil and freeze for about half an hour.
3. With your clean hands, shape the frozen mixture into small balls.

Place hazelnut-choco balls in an airtight container.

4. Munch and store the left overs the fridge.

Serves: 60

Calories: 151 per serving

Banana and Cherry Smoothie

Banana and Cherry a perfect flavor for a filling drink!

Ingredients

4 cups cherries, unsweetened

1 banana, chilled

4 cups green tea

½ cup prune juice

4 tbsp. yogurt

2 tbsp. chia seeds

Procedure

1. Mix all ingredients to a blender.

Add ice gradually as desired.

2. Blend until smooth.
3. Serve.

Serves: 2

Calories: 228 per serving

Rouge Flaxseed Smoothie

A no-sweat smoothie that you can prepare even on a day.

Ingredients

4 cups cherries, frozen and unsweetened

1 cup almonds. ground

1 cup freshly squeezed orange juice

4 tbsp. flaxseed

½ cup almonds, chopped

1 tsp. almond extract

Procedure

1. Put all ingredients except almonds in a food processor. Blend until smooth in texture.

Pour into choice of glass and sprinkle with almonds.

Serves: 4

Calories: 296 per serving

Chapter 18: Amazingly Clean Eating Recipes To Start Your Weight Loss

Since, you have plentiful knowledge of clean eating you must be needing clean eating recipes to get started with. So here come completely clean breakfast, lunch and dinner recipes to give you a great start. Enjoy scrumptious and healthy food prepared by you!

Day 1

Breakfast

Mixed Berries Milkshake

Yield: 1 serving
Preparation Time: 10 minutes

Ingredients

½ cup frozen blackberries
½ cup frozen strawberries
½ cup frozen blueberries
3 Medjool dates, pitted and chopped
¾ cup unsweetened almond milk

Procedure

1. In a high speed blender, add all ingredients and pulse till smooth.
2. Serve immediately.

Lunch

Beans & Corn Salad

Yield: 2 servings
Preparation Time: 15 minutes

Ingredients

¼ cup canned black beans, rinsed and drained
¼ cup canned red kidney beans, rinsed and drained
¼ cup corn kernels
¼ cup cherry tomatoes, halved
¼ cup avocado, peeled, pitted and cubed
2 cups romaine lettuce, torn
1 tablespoon fresh lemon juice
Salt and freshly ground black pepper, to taste

Procedure

1. In a serving bowl, add all ingredients and gently toss to coat well.
2. Serve immediately.

Dinner

Steak & Veggie Salad

Yield: 4 servings
Preparation Time: 20 minutes
Cooking Time: 6-10 minutes

Ingredients

1¾ pounds beef sirloin steak
Salt and freshly ground black pepper, to taste
1 large green bell pepper, seeded and sliced thinly
1 large carrot, peeled and sliced thinly
2 tomatoes, chopped
½ cup red onion, sliced
8 cups romaine lettuce
¼ cup extra-virgin olive oil

2 tablespoons fresh lemon juice
2 tablespoons red wine vinegar
1 teaspoon Worcestershire sauce
1 garlic clove, minced
2 tablespoons fresh cilantro, minced

Procedure

1. Preheat grill for high heat. Grease the grill grate.

Sprinkle the steak with a little salt and black pepper.

2. Grill for about 3-5 minutes from both sides or until desired doneness.
3. Transfer the steak onto a cutting board and let it cool.

With a sharp knife, cut the steak into desired slices.

4. In a large bowl, mix together bell pepper, carrot, tomato, onion and lettuce.
5. In a small bowl, add oil, lemon juice, vinegar, Worcestershire sauce, garlic, cilantro, salt and black pepper and beat till well combined.

Place steak over salad and drizzle with dressing.

6. Serve immediately.

Day 2

Breakfast

Creamy Healthy Smoothie

Yield: 1 serving
Preparation Time: 10 minutes

Ingredients

¼ of avocado, peeled, pitted and chopped
½ of banana, peeled and sliced
½ cup fresh blueberries
1 cup fresh spinach
¼ of cucumber, peeled and chopped
1½ teaspoons hemp seeds, shelled
¼ teaspoon wheatgrass powder
1 cup coconut water

Procedure

1. In a high speed blender, add all ingredients and pulse till smooth.
2. Serve immediately.

Lunch

Pasta & Veggie Salad

Yield: 10 servings
Preparation Time: 20 minutes
Cooking Time: 8-10 minutes

Ingredients

2 cups whole-wheat tri color rotini pasta
¼ cup balsamic vinegar
¼ cup extra-virgin olive oil
1 teaspoon raw honey
2 garlic cloves, minced
Salt and freshly ground black pepper, to taste
2 large carrots, peeled and chopped
1 large cucumber, peeled and chopped
1 cup celery, chopped
2 Roma tomatoes, chopped

1 red onion, chopped
2 scallions, chopped
2 tablespoons fresh cilantro, chopped
2 tablespoons fresh parsley, chopped

Procedure

1. In a large pan of lightly salted boiling water, add pasta and cook for about 8-10 minutes or according to package's directions.

Drain and rinse under cold water. Drain well and transfer into a large bowl.

2. In another bowl, add vinegar, oil, honey, garlic, salt and black pepper and beat till well combined.
3. Add dressing in the bowl with pasta. Add remaining ingredients and stir to combine.
4. Serve immediately.

Dinner

Chicken & Vegetables Soup

Yield: 4 servings
Preparation Time: 15 minutes
Cooking Time: 20 minutes

Ingredients

1 tablespoon extra-virgin olive oil
1 small carrot, peeled and chopped
½ cup onion, chopped
1 celery stalk, chopped
2 garlic cloves, minced
½ teaspoon ground cumin
¼ teaspoon red pepper flakes, crushed
1¼ cups zucchini, sliced

5 cups fat-free, low- sodium chicken broth
1¼ cups cooked chicken, chopped
2 cups fresh kale, trimmed and chopped
Salt and freshly ground black pepper, to taste
2 tablespoons fresh lime juice
2 tablespoons fresh cilantro, chopped

Procedure

1. In a large soup pan, heat oil on medium heat.
2. Add carrot, onion and celery and sauté for about 8-9 minutes.
3. Add garlic and spices and sauté for about 1 minute.
4. Add zucchini and broth and bring to a boil on high heat. Reduce the heat to medium-low.
5. Simmer for about 5 minutes.
6. Add cooked chicken and kale and simmer for about 5 minutes.
7. Stir in salt, black pepper and lime juice and remove from heat.
8. Serve hot with the garnishing of cilantro

Day 3

Breakfast

Feta Spinach Omelet

Yield:2 servings
Preparation Time: 15 minutes
Cooking Time:6½ minutes

Ingredients

4 large eggs
¼ cup cooked spinach, squeezed
2 scallions, chopped
2 tablespoons fresh parsley, chopped
½ cup feta cheese, crumbled

Freshly ground black pepper, to taste
2 teaspoons extra-virgin olive oil

Procedure

1. Preheat the broiler of oven. Arrange a rack about 4-inches from heating element.

In a bowl, crack the eggs and beat well.

2. Add remaining ingredients except oil and stir to combine.
3. In an ovenproof skillet, heat oil on medium heat.

Add egg mixture and tilt the skillet to spread the mixture evenly.

4. Immediately, reduce the heat to medium-low.
5. Cook for about 3-4 minutes or till golden brown.

Now, transfer the skillet under broiler and broil for about 1½-2½ minutes.

6. Cut the omelet into desired size wedges and serve.

Lunch

Green Veggies Soup

Yield: 4 servings
Preparation Time: 20 minutes
Cooking Time: 3-4 minutes

Ingredients

¼ cup almonds, soaked for overnight and drained
1 large avocado, peeled, pitted and chopped
½ small green bell pepper, seeded and chopped
2 cups fresh spinach leaves
1 small zucchini, chopped
2 celery stalks, chopped
2 tablespoons onion, chopped
1 garlic clove, chopped
½ cup fresh cilantro leaves
¼ cup fresh parsley leaves

2 tablespoons fresh lemon juice
Salt and freshly ground black pepper, to taste
2 cups vegetable fat-free, low- sodium broth

Procedure

1. In a high speed blender, add all ingredients and pulse till smooth.
2. Transfer the soup into a pan and cook on medium heat for 3-4 minutes or heated through.
3. Serve immediately.

Dinner

Noodles & Mixed Vegetables Soup

Yield: 4 servings
Preparation Time: 20 minutes
Cooking Time: 15 minutes

Ingredients

8-ounce whole wheat pasta (of your choice)
1 tablespoon extra-virgin olive oil
1 tablespoon fresh ginger, grated finely
1 jalapeño pepper, chopped
6-ounces fresh shiitake mushrooms, sliced thinly
¼ cup low-sodium soy sauce
4½ cups vegetable fat-free, low- sodium broth
3 carrots, peeled and julienned
6-ounce fresh green beans, trimmed and cut into 2-inch pieces
3 scallions, sliced

Procedure

1. In a large pan of lightly salted boiling water, cook the noodles for about 8-10 minutes or according to package's directions.
2. Drain well and keep aside.
3. Meanwhile in a large soup pan, heat oil on medium heat.

4. **Add ginger and jalapeño pepper and sauté for about 1 minute.**
5. Add mushrooms and cook for about 4-5 minutes.
6. Add soy sauce and broth and bring to a boil.
7. Stir in remaining vegetables and again bring to a boil.
8. Reduce the heat to medium-low.
9. Simmer for about 6-8 minutes or till desired doneness.
    10. Divide the noodles in 4 serving bowls
    11. Pour hot soup over noodles and serve immediately.

Day 4

Breakfast

Eggs with Vegetables

Yield:4 servings
Preparation Time: 15 minutes
Cooking Time:17 minutes

Ingredients

1 cup fresh green beans, trimmed and cut into 1-inch pieces
2 tablespoons extra-virgin olive oil
2 pounds boiling potatoes, sliced
2 garlic cloves, minced
1 jalapeño pepper, seeded and chopped
Pinch of red pepper flakes, crushed
Salt and freshly ground black pepper, to taste
4 eggs

Procedure

1. In a large pan of boiling water, add green beans and cook for about 3 minutes or till crisp.

Drain well and rinse under cold running water.

2. In a large nonstick skillet, heat oil on medium heat.
3. Place potato slices in the bottom of skillet in an even layer.

Cook for about 10-12 minutes, flipping occasionally.

4. Stir in remaining ingredients and except eggs.
5. Carefully, crack the eggs over veggie mixture.

Cover the skillet and cook for about 3-5 minutes.

6. Serve immediately.

Lunch

Tofu & Oats Burgers

Yield: 4 servings
Preparation Time: 15 minutes
Cooking Time: 16-20 minutes

Ingredients

1 pound firm tofu, pressed and crumbled
¾ cup rolled oats
¼ cup flaxseeds
2 cups frozen spinach, thawed and squeezed
1 medium onion, chopped finely
2 garlic cloves, minced
1 jalapeño pepper, seeded and minced
1 teaspoon ground cumin
½ teaspoon red pepper flakes, crushed
Salt and freshly ground black pepper, to taste
2 tablespoons extra-virgin olive oil
6 cups mixed fresh baby greens

Procedure

1. In a large bowl, mix together all ingredients except oil and salad greens. Keep aside for 10 minutes.

2. Make desired size patties from mixture.
3. In a nonstick frying pan, heat oil on medium heat.
4. **Cook patties for 8-10 minutes per side.**
5. Serve these patties with fresh greens.

Dinner

Tofu with Three Peas

Servings: 6
Preparation Time: 15 minutes
CookingTime: 18 minutes

Ingredients

1 tablespoon chile garlic sauce
3 tablespoons low-sodium soy sauce
2 tablespoonsextra-virgin olive oil, divided
1 (16-ounce) package extra-firm tofu, drained, pressed and cubed
1 cup onion, chopped
1 tablespoon fresh ginger, minced
2 garlic cloves, minced
1 cup frozen peas, thawed
2½ cups snow peas, trimmed
2½ cups sugar snap peas, trimmed

Procedure

1. In a bowl, mix together chile garlic sauce and soy sauce.
2. In a large skillet, heat 1 tablespoon of oil on medium-high heat.
3. Add tofu and cook, stirring occasionally for about 6-8 minutes or till browned completely.
4. **Transfer the tofu into a bowl**
5. In the same skillet, heat remaining oil on medium heat.
6. Add onion and sauté for about 3-4 minutes.
7. Add ginger and garlic and sauté for about 1 minute.

8. Stir in all three peas and cook for about 2-3 minutes.
9. Stir in sauce mixture and tofu and cook for about 1-2 minutes.
10. Serve hot.

Day 5

Breakfast

Bell Pepper Frittata

Yield:6 servings
Preparation Time: 15 minutes
Cooking Time:7 minutes

Ingredients

8 eggs
1 tablespoon fresh cilantro, chopped
1 tablespoon fresh basil, chopped
¼ teaspoon red pepper flakes, crushed
Salt and freshly ground black pepper, to taste
2 tablespoons extra-virgin olive oil
1 bunch scallions, chopped
1 cup red bell pepper, seeded and sliced thinly
½ cup goat cheese, crumbled

Procedure

1. Preheat the broiler of oven. Arrange a rack in upper third of oven.

In a bowl, add eggs, fresh herbs, red pepper flakes, salt and black pepper and beat well.

2. In an ovenproof skillet, heat oil on medium heat.
3. Add scallion and bell pepper and sauté for about 1 minute.

Add egg mixture over bell pepper mixture evenly and lift the edges to let the egg mixture flow underneath and cook for about 2-3 minutes.

4. Place the cheese on top in the form of dots.
5. Now, transfer the skillet under broiler and broil for about 2-3 minutes.
6. Cut the frittata into desired size slices and serve.

Lunch

Chicken Kebabs with Salad

Yield: 4 servings
Preparation Time: 15 minutes
Cooking Time: 6 minutes

Ingredients

For Kebabs:

1 teaspoon garlic, minced
1 tablespoon fresh thyme, minced
2 tablespoons fresh lemon juice
1 tablespoon extra-virgin olive oil
Salt and freshly ground black pepper, to taste
4 (6-ounce) skinless, boneless chicken breasts, cubed into ½-inch size

For Salad:

2 cups grape tomatoes, halved
1 red onion, chopped
6 cups lettuce leaves, torn
1 garlic clove, minced
2 tablespoons fresh cilantro, minced
2 tablespoons fresh lemon juice
2 tablespoons extra-virgin olive oil
Salt and freshly ground black pepper, to taste

Procedure

1. For chicken in a large bowl, mix together all ingredients except chicken cubes.
2. Add chicken cubes ant coat with marinade generously.
3. Cover and refrigerate to marinate for at least 2 hours.
4. **Preheat grill to high heat. Grease the grill grate.**
5. Remove the chicken from refrigerator and thread onto pre-soaked wooden skewers.
6. Grill for about 6-8 minutes, flipping occasionally or till desired doneness.
7. Meanwhile in a large bowl, mix together tomatoes, onion and lettuce.
8. In another bowl, add remaining ingredients and beat till well combined.
9. Pour dressing over salad and toss to coat.
10. Serve chicken kebabs with salad.

Dinner

Grilled Chicken Thighs

Yield: 4 servings
Preparation Time: 15 minutes
Cooking Time: 16 minutes

Ingredients

1 tablespoons fresh lime juice
½ tablespoon fresh thyme, minced
½ tablespoon fresh oregano, minced
½ teaspoon ground cumin
½ tablespoon red pepper flakes, crushed
¼ tablespoon paprika
1/8 teaspoon onion powder
1/8 teaspoon garlic powder
Salt and freshly ground black pepper, to taste
4 (4-ounce) skinless, boneless chicken thighs

For Serving:

8 cups fresh baby spinach

Procedure

1. Preheat the grill to medium-high heat. Grease the grill grate.

For chicken in a bowl, add all ingredients except chicken thighs and mix till well combined.

2. Coat the thighs with spice mixture generously.
3. Grill for about 8 minutes from both sides.

Serve the grilled thighs with spinach.

Day 6

Breakfast

Lemony Strawberry French Toasts

Yield: 2 servings
Preparation Time: 10 minutes
Cooking Time: 5 minutes

Ingredients

2 egg whites
½ teaspoon ground cinnamon
1½ teaspoons pure vanilla extract
2 grain-free bread slices
2 teaspoons butter
1 cup frozen strawberries
¼ teaspoon powdered stevia
3 teaspoons fresh lemon juice

Procedure

1. In a bowl, add egg whites, cinnamon and vanilla and beat well.

Add bread slices in the egg white mixture and coat from both sides evenly.

2. In a nonstick skillet, melt butter on medium heat.

3. Add slices and cook for about 5 minutes, flipping once in the middle way or till golden brown from both sides.

Meanwhile in a small nonstick pan, add strawberries on low heat.

4. Cook for about 2-3 minutes.
5. Stir in stevia lemon juice and remove from heat.
6. Top the French toasts with strawberry mixture and serve.

Lunch

Shrimp Rolls

Yield: 6 servings
Preparation Time: 20 minutes

Ingredients:

1-ounce cellophane noodles

1 tablespoon white vinegar

6 spring roll wrappers

12 medium cooked shrimp, peeled, deveined and halved lengthwise

2 medium carrots, peeled and julienned

½ cup green cabbage, shredded

½ cup red cabbage, shredded

1 medium seedless cucumber, julienned

1 avocado, peeled, pitted and sliced

1 head Boston lettuce, torn

2 tablespoons fresh cilantro, chopped

2 tablespoons fresh basil, chopped

Procedure

1. In a pan of boiling water, place cellophane and keep aside for 10 minutes.
2. Drain well and transfer into a bowl.
3. Add vinegar and toss to coat and keep aside.
4. In a large round pie plate, pour hot water. Place the each wrapper for about for 15-30 seconds or till soft.
5. Meanwhile in a large bowl, mix together remaining all ingredients.
6. Place each wrapper onto a large piece of parchment paper.
7. Divide shrimp mixture over the center of wrapper evenly, leaving at least an inch on the sides.
8. Carefully, fold the bottom edge of wrapper over the filling and roll tightly.
9. Secure each wrap with toothpick and serve.

Dinner

Veggie Stuffed Chicken Breasts

Yield: 8 servings
Preparation Time: 15 minutes
Cooking Time: 12 minutes

Ingredients:

1 large red bell pepper, seeded and chopped finely
2 tablespoons kalamata olives, pitted and chopped finely
1 tablespoon fresh parsley, minced
¼ cup feta cheese, crumbled
8 (6-ounce) skinless, boneless chicken breast halves
Salt and freshly ground black pepper, to taste

Procedure

1. Preheat grill for medium-high heat. Grease the grill grate.

In a bowl, mix together all ingredients except chicken breasts and seasoning.

2. With a sharp knife, make a horizontal slit in each breast half to form a pocket.
3. Fill each pocket with vegetable mixture evenly and secure with toothpicks.

Sprinkle with salt and black pepper evenly,

4. Grill for about 6 minutes from both sides or till desired doneness.

Day 7

Breakfast

Fruity Oat Muffins

Yield: 5 servings
Preparation Time: 15 minutes
Cooking Time: 12 minutes

Ingredients:

½ cup rolled oats
¼ cup almond flour
½ teaspoon baking soda
2 tablespoons flaxseeds
½ teaspoon ground cinnamon
Pinch of ground nutmeg
1 egg
¼ cup unsalted butter, softened
2 tablespoons banana, peeled and sliced
½ teaspoon vanilla extract
¼ cup fresh blueberries

Procedure

1. Preheat the oven to 375 degrees F. Grease 10 cups of a muffin tray.
2. In a blender, add all ingredients except blueberries and pulse till smooth and creamy.
3. Transfer the mixture into a bowl and gently, fold in blueberries.
4. **Transfer the mixture into prepared muffin cups evenly.**
5. Bake for about 10-12 minutes or till a toothpick inserted in the center comes out clean.

Lunch

Lemony Quinoa & Green Beans

Yield: 4 servings
Preparation Time: 10 minutes
Cooking Time: 20 minutes

Ingredients:

2 tablespoons extra-virgin olive oil, divided
1 small onion, chopped
2 garlic cloves, minced
1 Serrano pepper, seeded and chopped finely
1 cup quinoa
Salt and freshly ground black pepper, to taste
1¾ cups fat-free, low-sodium vegetable broth
1 pound fresh green beans, trimmed and cut into 2-inch pieces
2 tablespoons fresh lemon juice

Procedure

1. In a pan, heat 1 tablespoon of oil on medium heat.
2. Add onion and sauté for about 2-3 minutes.
3. Add garlic and Serrano pepper and sauté for about 1 minute.

4. Add quinoa and cook, stirring continuously for about 1 minute.
5. Add salt, black pepper and broth and bring to a boil.
6. Reduce the heat to low. Cover and simmer for about 15 minutes.
7. Remove from heat and keep aside, covered for about 10 minutes. With a fork, fluff the quinoa.
8. Meanwhile in a pan of salted boiling water, add beans and cook for about 4-5 minutes or till crisp tender.
9. In a large serving bowl, mix together quinoa and green beans. Sprinkle with a little salt and black pepper.
10. Drizzle with lemon juice and remaining oil and serve.

Dinner

Simple Grilled Beef Steak

Yield: 8 servings
Preparation Time: 15 minutes
Cooking Time: 8-10 minutes

Ingredients

4 (½-pound) grass-fed beef top sirloin steaks
2 tablespoons extra-virgin olive oil
2 tablespoons steak seasoning

Procedure

1. Preheat the grill for high heat. Grease the grill grate.

In a large bowl, mix together oil and seasoning mix and coat the steaks with mixture generously.

2. Grill the steak for about 4-5 minutes per side or till desired doneness.
3. Cut each steak in half and serve.

Day 8

Breakfast

Baked Cherry Pancakes

Yield: 4 servings
Preparation Time: 15 minutes
Cooking Time: 15-20 minutes

Ingredients

1 teaspoon unsalted butter
½ cup whole-wheat pastry flour
1/8 teaspoon ground cinnamon
Pinch of salt
3 eggs
½ cup fat-free milk
1 tablespoon unsalted butter, melted
1 teaspoon vanilla extract
2 cups fresh sweet cherries, pitted and halved
¼ cup almonds, chopped

Procedure

1. Preheat the oven to 450 degrees F.

In a 10-inch ovenproof skillet, add 1 teaspoon of butter and place the skillet into oven.

2. In a bowl, mix together flour, cinnamon and salt.
3. In another bowl, add eggs, milk, butter and vanilla and beat till well combined.

Add egg mixture into flour mixture and mix till well combined.

4. Remove the skillet from oven and tilt to spread the melted butter evenly.
5. Place cherries in the bottom of skillet in a single layer.

Place the flour mixture over cherries evenly

Top with almonds evenly.

6. Bake for about 15-20 minutes or till a toothpick inserted in the center comes out clean.
7. Remove from oven and let it cool for at least 5 minutes before slicing.
8. Cut into 4 equal sized wedges and serve.

Lunch

Spinach & Tofu Stir Fry

Yield: 2 servings
Preparation Time: 10 minutes
Cooking Time: 15 minutes

Ingredients

2 tablespoons extra-virgin olive oil
1 medium onion, chopped
2 garlic cloves, minced
2 teaspoons fresh basil, chopped
½ pound firm tofu, pressed and cubed
4 cups fresh spinach, chopped
Salt and freshly ground black pepper, to taste
1 tablespoon fresh lemon juice

Procedure

1. In a large skillet, heat oil on medium heat.
2. Add onion and sauté for about 3-4 minutes.
3. Add garlic and basil and sauté for about 1 minute.
4. **Add tofu and stir fry for about 5-6 minutes.**
5. Add spinach, salt and black pepper and stir fry for about 3-4 minutes.
6. Stir in lemon juice and remove from heat.
7. Serve hot.

Dinner

Pork with Bok Choy

Yield: 4 servings
Preparation Time: 15 minutes
Cooking Time: 18 minutes

Ingredients

1 tablespoon extra-virgin olive oil
4 scallions, chopped
2 garlic cloves, minced
2 tablespoons fresh ginger, minced
1 Serrano pepper, chopped finely
1 pound pork loin steaks, trimmed and cut into strips
3 tablespoons low-sodium soy sauce
½ pound bokchoy, sliced

Procedure

1. In a large skillet, heat oil on medium heat.

Add scallion and sauté for about 2 minutes.

2. Add garlic, ginger and Serrano pepperand sauté for about 1 minute.
3. Add pork and cook for about 8-10 minutes or till tender.

Add soy sauce and bok choy and cook for about 4-5 minutes.

4. Serve hot.

Day 9
Breakfast

Quinoa & Date Bowl

Yield: 4 servings
Preparation Time: 10 minutes
Cooking Time: 10-15 minutes

Ingredients

2 cups unsweetened almond milk
1 cup quinoa
¼ teaspoon vanilla extract
Pinch of ground cinnamon
2 Medjool dates, pitted and chopped very finely
1 cup fresh strawberries, hulled and sliced

Procedure

1. In a pan, mix together milk, quinoa, vanilla and cinnamon on low heat.

Cook, stirring occasionally for about 10-15 minutes.

2. Stir in chopped dates and immediately, remove from heat.
3. Serve with the garnishing of strawberries.

Lunch

Broth Braised Cabbage

Yield: 4 servings
Preparation Time: 15 minutes
Cooking Time: 25 minutes

Ingredients

1½ teaspoons extra-virgin olive oil
2 garlic cloves, minced
3 cups green cabbage, chopped
1 onion, sliced thinly
1 cup fat-free, low- sodium vegetable broth
Salt and freshly ground black pepper, to taste

Procedure

1. In a large nonstick skillet, heat oil on high heat.

Add garlic and sauté for about1 minute.
2. Add cabbage and onion and sauté for about 3-4 minutes.
3. Stir in broth, salt and black pepper and immediately, reduce the heat to low.

Cover and cook for about 20 minutes.
4. Serve warm.

Dinner

Grilled Lamb Chops & Veggies

Yield: 8 servings
Preparation Time: 15 minutes
Cooking Time: 15 minutes

Ingredients

For Chops:

¼ cup balsamic vinegar
3 tablespoons extra-virgin olive oil
2 tablespoons fresh lemon juice
4 minced garlic cloves
2 teaspoons dried rosemary, crushed
Salt and freshly ground black pepper, as required
8 (1-inch thick) lamb chops

ForVeggies:

32 fresh cherry tomatoes, stemmed
1½ pounds asparagus, trimmed
2 tablespoons olive oil
2 teaspoons minced fresh parsley
2 teaspoons minced freshrosemary
Salt and freshly ground black pepper, as required

Procedure

1. In a large bowl, mix together oil, vinegar, lemon juice, garlic, rosemary, salt and black pepper.

Add chops and coat with marinade generously. Cover and refrigerate to marinate for about 4-5 hours.

2. Remove from refrigerator and keep in room temperature for at least 30 minutes.
3. Preheat the grill to medium-high heat. Grease the grill grate.

Cook the chops for about 4 minutes per side.

4. Transfer the chops into a large plate. Cover with foil paper to keep them warm.
5. Meanwhile for vegetables in a large bowl, add all ingredients and toss to coat well.

Thread the cherry tomatoes onto presoaked wooden skewers.

After removing chops from grill, grease the grill grate again.

6. Grill the tomatoes for about 3-4 minutes per side.
7. Now, increase the temperature of grill to high heat.
8. Grill the asparagus for about 2-3 minutes.
9. Divide the chops, tomatoes and asparagus in 8 serving plates evenly and serve.

Day 10

Breakfast

Nutty Oatmeal

Yield: 4 servings
Preparation Time: 10 minutes
Cooking Time: 3-4 minutes

Ingredients

1 cup steel cut oats
2 cups unsweetened almond milk, divided
4-6 drops liquid stevia

1 large banana, peeled and sliced
¼ cup walnuts, chopped

Procedure

1. In a bowl, add oats, 1 cup of milk and stevia and stir well.

Cover and refrigerate for at least overnight.

2. Remove from refrigerator. Transfer the oats mixture into a pan on medium heat.
3. Add remaining milk and stir to combine.

Cook for 3-4 minutes or till heated completely.

4. Transfer oat mixture into serving bowls.
5. Top with banana slices and walnuts and serve.

Lunch

Shrimp in Sweet & Sour Sauce

Yield: 2 servings
Preparation Time: 15 minutes
Cooking Time: 10 minutes

Ingredients

For Sauce:

3 tablespoons fresh orange juice
1 tablespoon organic honey
1 tablespoon low-sodium soy sauce
½ tablespoon balsamic vinegar

For Shrimp:

¾ pound shrimp, peeled and deveined
½ tablespoons arrowroot powder
1 tablespoon extra-virgin olive oil
2 garlic cloves, minced
1 teaspoon fresh ginger, minced

Procedure

1. In a bowl, mix together all sauce ingredients. Keep aside.

In a bowl, add shrimp and sprinkle with arrowroot powder and toss to coat well.

2. In a large skillet, heat oil on medium-high heat.
3. Add garlic and ginger and sauté for about 1 minute.

Add shrimp and cook for about 3 minutes.

4. Add sauce and cook, stirring continuously for about 2 minutes.
5. With a slotted spoon, transfer the shrimp into a bowl.

Cook, stirring for about 2-4 minutes or till desired thickness.

6. Serve shrimp with the topping of sauce.

Dinner

Salmon & Veggie Parcel

Yield: 6 servings
Preparation Time: 15 minutes
Cooking Time: 20 minutes

Ingredients

6 (3-ounce) salmon fillets
Salt and freshly ground black pepper, to taste
1 yellow bell pepper, seeded and sliced thinly
1 red bell pepper, seeded and sliced thinly
4 plum tomatoes, sliced thinly
1 small onion, sliced thinly
½ cup fresh parsley, chopped
1/3 cup capers
¼ cup extra-virgin olive oil
2 tablespoons fresh lemon juice

Procedure

1. Preheat the oven to 400 degrees F.

Arrange 6 foil pieces of foil paper on smooth surface.
2. Place 1 salmon fillet on each foil paper. Sprinkle with salt and black pepper.
3. In a bowl, mix together bell peppers, tomato and onion.

Place veggie mixture over each fillet evenly.
4. Top with parsley and capers evenly.
5. Drizzle with oil and lemon juice.

Fold the foil paper around salmon mixture to seal it.

Arrange the foil packets onto a large baking sheet in a single layer.
6. Bake for about 20 minutes.

Conclusion

Thank you again for downloading this book!

I hope this book was able to help you to understand the how's and why's of eating cleaner and greener, and the impact that even just a few dietary changes can have on your life and our world.

The next step is to revise your grocery list, read a lot of labels ... then start eating cleaner!

Part 2

Parsley Potatoes

Ingredients:

Potatoes:

3-4 red or baby Idaho potatoes, cut into quarters

½ Tbsp. extra-virgin olive oil

¼ tsp. garlic powder

¼ tsp. onion powder

¼ tsp. kosher salt

Pinch of pepper

Tomato-Parsley Reduction Sauce:

1 tsp. extra-virgin olive oil

½ clove garlic, minced

1 Tbsp. diced onion

1 can (5.5 oz.) tomato juice

½ tsp. cornstarch

¾ tsp. horseradish

½ Tbsp. ketchup

¼ tsp. celery seed

¼ tsp. paprika

½ Tbsp. lemon juice

A few dashes of hot sauce, to taste

Salt & Pepper, to taste

¼ cup parsley, chopped

Directions

Preheat the oven to 400 degrees F and line a baking sheet with parchment paper.

Combine quartered potatoes with the olive oil and spices listed in the first section.

Transfer potatoes to prepared baking sheet and spread out evenly. Bake for 35-40 minutes, flipping the potatoes every 10 minutes or so to ensure even crisping.

While the potatoes are roasting, heat olive oil in a saucepan over medium heat. Add garlic and onion; cook, stirring often, for about 3-5 minutes, or until translucent.

In a separate bowl, whisk together tomato juice, cornstarch, horseradish, ketchup, celery, seed, paprika, lemon juice and hot sauce until well-combined.

Add the tomato mixture to the saucepan with the garlic and onion. Cook 10-15 minutes, stirring occasionally--the mixture will thicken and reduce by almost half. Add salt and pepper to taste.

Drizzle the tomato reduction over the roasted potatoes and top with chopped parsley.

Nutritional Information

Calories: 350

Total Fat: 4.4g

Saturated Fat: 0.2g

Carbohydrates: 73g

Protein: 4.6g

Wild Rice Chowder

Ingredients:

¼ cup raw cashews, soaked overnight and drained

½ medium potato, cooked with skin

½ can white beans, rinsed

1 tsp. extra-virgin olive oil

½ yellow onion, diced

2 cloves garlic, minced

½ rib celery, diced

¼ cup wild rice, not cooked

¼ cup brown rice, soaked overnight and drained

2 cups vegetable broth (or water)

¼ Tbsp. white or yellow miso paste

1 Tbsp. white balsamic vinegar (or ½ Tbsp. lemon juice)

¼ cup white wine (optional)

Salt & Pepper, to taste

¼ cup fresh parsley, chopped

Directions:

Combine cashews, cooked potato, and white beans in a food processor or blender and blend well until completely smooth. If needed, add a little of the water or vegetable broth to blend.

Heat oil in a large saucepan or small pot over medium heat. Add the onion, garlic, and celery and a pinch of salt. Stir and continue cooking until soft, about 3-5 minutes.

Add the wild rice and brown rice. Stir and cook for another 1-2 minutes

Add the vegetable broth and bring the mixture to a boil. Once it boils, reduce the heat to medium.

Whisk the miso with a bit of water to thin it out. Add the miso, vinegar, white wine and a pinch of pepper.

Stir in the cashew mixture and continue to cook the soup at a steady simmer, stirring frequently to ensure the rice does not stick to the bottom. Add more broth if you would like a thinner chowder.

Simmer for 30-45 minutes (until the wild rice is cooked).

Season with salt and pepper and top with parsley. Any extra can be stored in an airtight container, in the fridge, for up to a week.

Nutritional Information (for one serving, approximately 1/4th of soup)

Calories: 175.1

Total Fat: 4.3g

Saturated Fat: 0.9g

Carbohydrates: 28.7g

Protein: 5.4g

Vegan Bean Burger

Ingredients:

1 Tbsp. onion, diced

1 Tbsp. grated carrot

1 Tbsp. bread crumbs

1/4 cup kidney beans, rinsed and drained

¼ cup cannellini beans, rinsed and drained

½ Tbsp. parsley, finely chopped

Pinch of chili powder

Salt and Pepper to taste

1 tsp. flour

3 Tbsp. Extra Virgin Olive Oil for frying

Whole wheat hamburger bun

Directions:

Put half the breadcrumbs in a mixing bowl.

Heat 1 Tbsp. olive oil in a medium saucepan and add onion. Cook for 3 minutes, or until softened and then add the grated carrot and cook for an additional 2-3 minutes. Add onions and carrots the breadcrumbs.

In a separate bowl, roughly mash the kidney and cannellini beans with a fork and then stir into the carrot mixture. Add a pinch of chili powder, salt and pepper.

In a shallow bowl, combine the remaining breadcrumbs with flour, parsley, salt, and pepper.

Shape your bean-carrot blend into 1 or 2 burger patties. Thoroughly coat the patty in the flour mixture.

Heat 2 Tbsp. olive oil in a frying pan over medium heat. Carefully add your burger patty and fry each side until golden brown (about 5 minutes).

Place in whole wheat bun, top with desired condiments, and enjoy.

Nutritional Information

Calories: 225.2

Total Fat: 1.6g

Saturated Fat: 0.2g

Carbohydrates: 44.7g

Protein: 8g

Chard with Garbanzo Beans and Couscous

Ingredients:

4 Tbsp. couscous

2 Tbsp. pine nuts

1 Tbsp. Extra Virgin Olive Oil

1 clove garlic, thinly sliced

5 Tbsp. garbanzo beans, drained and rinsed

2 Tbsp. golden raisins (or dark)

½ bunch Swiss Chard, stems trimmed

Salt and Pepper, to taste

Directions:

Place the couscous in a large bowl and add 1/3 cup boil water. Stir, cover tightly and let stand for 10 minutes.

While the couscous cooks, toast the pine nuts in a large skillet over low heat. Toast for 3-4 minutes, shaking the pan frequently. Set toasted pine nuts aside.

Heat olive oil in the skillet over medium heat. Add the garlic and cook until fragrant, about 1 minute.

Add the garbanzo beans, raisins, chard, salt and pepper. Cook for about 5 minutes, stirring occasionally, until chard is tender. Remove from heat.

Fluff couscous with a fork and place in a bowl or plate. Top with prepared chard, sprinkle with pine nuts, and enjoy.

Nutritional Information

Calories: 142.4

Total Fat: 6 g

Saturated Fat: 0.25 g

Carbohydrates: 17.8 g

Protein: 4.3 g

Garbanzo Curry

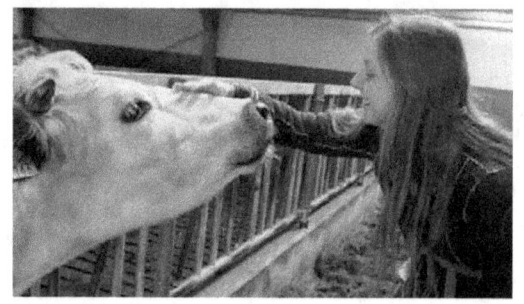

Ingredients:

¾ tsp. extra-virgin olive oil

¼ onion, minced

½ clove garlic, minced

¼ tsp. fresh ginger root, finely chopped

1 whole clove

1/8 tsp. cinnamon

1/8 tsp. ground cumin

1/8 tsp ground coriander.

Pinch of salt

1/8 tsp. cayenne pepper

1/8 tsp. ground turmeric

¼ 15oz-can garbanzo beans, drained and rinsed.

2 Tbsp. chopped fresh cilantro

1/4 cup jasmine rice

1/2 cup water

Directions:

First prepare the rice by placing both the rice and water in a medium saucepan or small pot. Turn the heat to high until it begins to boil, and then reduce to low, cover and let simmer for 15 minutes.

Heat olive oil in a large frying pan over medium heat for 1 minute. Sauté onions until tender, about 3-4 minutes.

Stir in garlic, ginger, clove, cinnamon, cumin, coriander, salt, cayenne, and turmeric. Cook for 1 minute over medium heat, stirring constantly.

Add in garbanzo beans and a little bit of water (about ½ Tbsp.).

Continue to cook for, stirring occasionally, for about 15-20 minutes, or until all the ingredients are well-blended and cooked through. Remove from heat.

Place cooked rice in a bowl, top with garbanzo curry, and garnish with cilantro.

Nutritional Information

Calories: 294.9

Total Fat: 4.5g

Saturated Fat: 0.7g

Carbohydrates: 56.5g

Protein: 7.1g

Vegan Polenta

Ingredients:

1/4 (8 oz.) container of tofu, drained

1/4 (16oz) tube prepared polenta

1/2 Tbsp. Extra virgin olive oil

1/2 banana, sliced lengthwise

1/4 cup black beans, undrained

1/2 avocado, sliced thinly

1/4 mango, diced

1 Tbsp. diced onion

1/4 jalapeno, seeded and diced

Salt and pepper, to taste

Directions:

Preheat the oven's broiler and set the oven rack about 6 inches from the heat source.

Slice the tofu and polenta into equal-sized slabs, brush with olive oil and arrange on a greased baking sheet.

Cook the tofu and polenta under the broiler until the tops are crispy, about 5 minutes. Remove from onion and set aside.

Heat the olive oil in medium skillet over medium-high heat. Sauté the bananas until crispy on the outside, about 5 minutes. Remove from oil and set aside.

Place the black beans into a blender and blend until it becomes a thick sauce.

In a separate bowl, combine mango, onion, jalapeno, salt and pepper.

To arrange, place a slice of polenta on a plate and top with 1/4 of the bean sauce, then tofu, banana, avocado, and then top with the mango salsa and serve.

Nutritional Information
Calories: 409.9
Total Fat: 15.5 g
Saturated Fat: 4.6 g
Carbohydrates: 54 g
Protein: 13.6 g

Ginger Stir-Fry with Coconut Rice

Ingredients:
1/2 tsp. corn starch
1/2 clove garlic, crushed
1/2 tsp. chopped fresh ginger root, divided
2 tsp. extra virgin olive-oil, divided
1/4 cup broccoli florets
1 Tbsp. snow peas
2 Tbsp. julienned carrots

1 Tbsp. red bell pepper, diced

1 tsp. soy sauce

1 tsp. water

1/2 Tbsp. chopped onion

1/4 cup jasmine rice

1/4 cup coconut milk

1/4 cup water

Sriracha (or other hot sauce)

Directions:

First prepare the rice by placing the rice, coconut milk, and water in a medium saucepan or small pot. Turn the heat to high until it begins to boil, and then reduce to low, cover and let simmer for 15 minutes, or until most of the coconut milk has been absorbed.

In a large bowl, blend cornstarch, garlic, half the ginger, and 1 tsp. olive oil until cornstarch is dissolved.

Add the broccoli, snow peas, carrots, and bell pepper, tossing to lighting coat.

Heat the remaining olive oil in a wok over medium heat. Add vegetables, cook for 1 minute, stirring constantly to prevent burning.

Add onions, salt, remaining ginger, soy sauce and water. Cook until vegetables are tender, but still crisp—about 2 minutes.

Place coconut rice in a bowl, top with ginger stir fry. Add Sriracha to taste.

Nutritional Information

Calories: 338.6

Total Fat: 16.2 g

Saturated Fat: 13.1 g

Carbohydrates: 42 g

Protein: 6.2 g

Avocado Tacos

Ingredients:

1 avocado, peeled, pitted, and mashed

2 Tbsp. onions, diced

1/8 tsp. garlic salt

1 tsp. lemon juice

Drizzle olive oil

2 Tbsp. tomato, diced

2 tsp. cilantro, chopped

Salt and pepper, to taste

1/4 cup black beans, drained and rinsed

1/2 garlic clove, chopped

Salt and pepper, to taste

Directions:

Preheat oven to 325 degrees F.

In a medium saucepan, heat olive oil over medium heat and add the garlic and half the onions and cook until translucent, about 2-5 minutes.

Add the black beans, turn heat the low. Stir occasionally and allow the beans to heat while you work on the filling.

Arrange corn tortillas in a single layer on a large baking sheet, and place in the preheated oven 2 to 5 minutes, until heated through.

In a medium bowl, mix avocado, remaining onion, tomatoes, garlic salt, pepper, lemon juice and a drizzle of olive oil.

Spread tortillas with avocado mixture, add black beans and top with cilantro.

Nutritional Information
Calories: 377.1
Total Fat: 18.3 g
Saturated Fat: 3.4g
Carbohydrates: 43.8 g
Protein: 9.3 g

Vegan Style Shepherd's Pie

Ingredients:
Mashed potatoes:
5 russet potatoes, peeled and cut into 1-inch cubes
1/2 cup vegan mayonnaise
1/2 cup soy milk (or other milk substitute)
1/4 cup olive oil
3 Tbsp. vegan cream cheese
2 tsp. salt
Filling:
2 carrots, diced

2 stalks celery, diced

3/4 cup broccoli florets

1 tsp. Italian seasoning

1 clove garlic, minced

1/2 tsp. celery seed (optional)

Pepper, to taste

1 (14 oz.) package vegan ground beef substitute

1 Tbsp. extra virgin olive oil

1 large yellow onion, diced

1/2 cup Cheddar-style soy cheese, shredded

Directions:

Place potatoes in a large pot, cover with cold water, and bring to a boil over medium-high heat. Turn the heat to medium-low and simmer the potatoes until tender, about 25 minutes. Drain and return to the pot.

In a bowl, combine the vegan mayonnaise, soy milk, olive oil, vegan cream cheese, and salt. Add to the potatoes mix with a potato masher until smooth and fluffy. Set aside.

Preheat the oven to 400 degrees F and grease a 2-quart baking dish.

In a medium skillet, heat the olive oil over medium heat. Add the onions, carrots, celery, and broccoli and cook for 10 minutes, or until softened. Stir in the Italian seasoning, celery seed, garlic, and pepper.

Reduce the heat to medium-low and crumble the vegan ground beef substitute into the skillet. Cook and stir, until the mixture is hot, about 5 minutes.

Spread the vegetable and "meat" filling into the bottom of the baking dish, and top with the mashed potatoes, smoothing them into an even layer. Top the whole pie with the shredded soy cheese.

Bake in a preheated oven until the cheese is melted and slightly browned, approximately 20 minutes. Remove and serve. Leftovers can be stored in an airtight container, in the fridge, for up to a week.

Nutritional Information (for $1/6^{th}$ of the pie)

Calories: 558.4

Total Fat: 24.4 g

Saturated Fat: 3.6 g

Carbohydrates: 64.5 g

Protein: 20.2 g

BBQ Tempeh Sandwiches:

Ingredients:

1/4 cup barbeque sauce, any kind

1/4 (8 oz.) package tempeh, crumbled

3/4 tsp. extra virgin olive oil

1/4 red bell pepper, seeded and diced

1/4 green bell pepper, seeded and diced

1/4 red onion, diced

1 Kaiser roll, split and toasted

Directions:

Pour the barbeque sauce into a medium bowl and crumble the tempeh into the sauce. Stir until the tempeh is covered, and let marinate for at least 10 minutes.

Heat olive oil in a skillet over medium heat. Add the onion, red, and green bell peppers. Cook for 4-5 minutes, stirring frequently.

Add the tempeh and barbeque sauce, stir and let cook until tempeh is heated through, about 8-10 minutes.

Spoon the bbq tempeh mixture into the toasted Kaiser roll and serve.

Nutritional Information

Calories: 383.1

Total Fat: 11.5g

Saturated Fat: 2.1g

Carbohydrates: 54.7g

Protein: 15.2g

Vegan Pasta with Pine Nuts

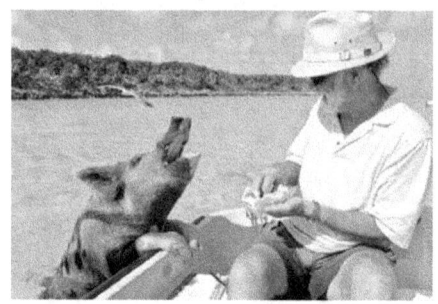

Ingredients:

1/2 cup farfalle pasta

1 roma tomato, diced

1 Tbsp. extra virgin olive oil

1 clove garlic, minced

2 Tbsp. fresh basil, cut into thin strips

Salt and pepper, to taste

2 Tbsp. pine nuts

Directions:

Bring a small pot of salted water to a boil. Add pasta and cook for 8-10 minutes. Drain.

In a large bowl, gently toss the cooked pasta, tomatoes, olive oil, garlic and basil.

Season with salt and pepper and top with pine nuts.

Nutritional Information
Calories: 275.6
Total Fat: 14.8 g
Saturated Fat:1.2 g
Carbohydrates: 32.2 g
Protein: 3.4 g

Mediterranean Zucchini

Ingredients:

1 tsp. extra virgin olive oil

2 Tbsp. onion, diced

2 Tbsp. red bell pepper, diced

1 clove garlic, diced

1/4 cup whole peeled tomatoes, chopped

1/2 cup finely chopped zucchini

1/4 cup cannellini beans, drained

Pinch oregano

Salt and pepper, to taste

1/4 cup rice, any kind

1/2 cup water

Directions:

First prepare the rice by placing the rice and water in a medium saucepan or small pot. Turn the heat to high until it begins to boil, and then reduce to low, cover and let simmer for 15 minutes, or until all the water has been absorbed.

Heat oil in a small saucepan over medium heat. Stir in onion, red bell pepper, and garlic and cook until fragrant, about 2-5 minutes.

Add tomatoes, zucchini, oregano, salt and pepper. Reduce heat, cover, and simmer for 20 minutes, stirring occasionally.

Stir in the cannellini beans into the zucchini mixture and continue cooking for 10 minutes.

Spoon over the cooked rice and serve.

Nutritional Information
Calories: 292.3
Total Fat: 7.5g
Saturated Fat: 0.9g
Carbohydrates: 47.2g
Protein: 9g

Pumpkin-Apple Curry

Ingredients:

1/3 cup red lentils

1/3 cup brown lentils

2 1/2 cups water

1/8 tsp turmeric

1 tsp. extra virgin olive oil

1/4 onion, diced

3 tomatoes, diced

1 clove garlic, minced

2 tsp. curry powder

3/4 tsp. ground cumin

1/8 tsp. salt

1/8 tsp. black pepper

1/8 tsp. ground cloves

2/3 cup peeled and seeded pumpkin, cut into 1-inch cubes

1/2 potato, diced

1 carrot, diced

1 Granny smith apple, cored and diced

Directions:

Place the red and brown lentils in a pan with the water and turmeric. Cook over medium-low heat until tender, about 45 minutes. Drain, and reserve 1 cup of the cooking liquid.

In a medium pot, heat the oil over medium heat. Stir in the onion, cook until translucent, about 5 minutes. Add in the tomatoes and garlic, cook for 5 minutes, stirring occasionally.

Mix in the curry powder, cumin, salt, pepper, and cloves. Add the cooked lentils, reserved cooking liquid, pumpkin, potatoes, and carrots. Cover and cook over medium-low heat for 35-45 minutes, or until the vegetables are tender.

Stir in the apple and lentils. Cook for an additional 15 minutes.

Nutritional Information

Calories: 199.8

Total Fat: 3.4 g

Saturated Fat: 0.1 g

Carbohydrates: 32.3 g

Protein: 10.1 g

Garlic-Ginger Tofu

Ingredients:

1 tsp. extra virgin olive oil

1 garlic clove, minced

2 tsp. minced fresh ginger root

Squeeze of lime juice

1/2 tsp. tamari

1/4 pound firm tofu

1/4 rice, any variety

1/2 cup of water

Directions:

First prepare the rice by placing the rice and water in a medium saucepan or small pot. Turn the heat to high until it begins to boil, and then reduce to low, cover and let simmer for 15 minutes, or until all the water has been absorbed.

Drain tofu with a paper toil and pat dry. Cut into cubes.

Heat oil in a wok over medium heat. Stir in garlic and ginger, cook for 1 minute.

Add tofu to the pan with tamari, and stir to coat. Cover and continue cooking for 20 minutes.

Serve tofu over rice and top with a squeeze of lime juice.

Nutritional Information

Calories: 243.1

Total Fat: 3.9g

Saturated Fat: 1g

Carbohydrates: 36 g

Protein: 6g

Baked Potato with Lentils

Ingredients:

1 tsp. extra virgin olive oil

1/2 white onion, halved and sliced into rings

1 garlic clove, minced

1/4 cup lentils

1 cup water

1/2 tsp. salt

1/2 tsp. cumin

Black pepper, to taste

1 clove garlic, crushed

1 russet potato

Drizzle of olive oil

Directions:

First prepare the baked potato. Preheat the oven to 400 degrees F. Wash the potato and then pierce a few times with a fork, and place it directly on rack in preheated oven and cook for 45 minutes. Place a baking sheet on the rack below to catch any drippings. Once cooked, remove from oven and set aside.

Heat olive oil in a heavy pan over medium heat. Sauté the onion for 5 minutes or until it begins to turn golden. Add minced garlic and sauté for another minute.

Add lentils and water to the saucepan. Bring the mixture to a boil, then cover, lower the heat, and simmer for 35 minutes, or until the lentils are soft.

Add the salt, cumin, and crushed garlic clove to the mixture. Cover and simmer until all is heater and integrated, about 10 minutes.

Cut open the baked potato, drizzle with olive oil, and fill with the lentil mixture. Season with salt and pepper and serve.

Nutritional Information

Calories: 241.5

Total Fat: 4.3g

Saturated Fat: 0.2g

Carbohydrates: 41 g

Protein: 9.7 g

Vegan Mac and No-Cheese

Ingredients:

¾ cup uncooked elbow macaroni

1 tsp. extra virgin olive oil

2 Tbsp. onion, chopped

1 garlic clove, chopped

¼ cup cashews

1 Tbsp. lemon juice

1/3 cup water

Salt and pepper, to taste

1 Tbsp. extra virgin olive oil

2 Tbsp. roasted red peppers, drained

½ tsp. garlic powder

½ tsp. onion powder

Directions:

Preheat oven to 350 degrees F.

Bring a medium pot of salted water to a boil. Add pasta and cook for 8 to 10 minutes. Drain and transfer to a small baking dish.

Heat olive oil in a medium saucepan over medium heat. Stir in onion and garlic and cook until fragrant and lightly browned, about 3-5 minutes. Add to the macaroni.

Using a blender or food processor, combine cashews, lemon juice, water and a pinch of salt. Gradually add in 1 Tbsp. olive oil, roasted red peppers, garlic powder and onion powder. Blend until smooth. Mix thoroughly with the macaroni.

Bake for 45 minutes in the preheated oven, or until slightly browned on top. Allow to cool 10-15 minutes, top with black pepper and serve.

Nutritional Information
Calories: 206.6
Total Fat: 9.8 g
Saturated Fat: 0.3g
Carbohydrates: 25.5 g
Protein: 4.1 g

Soba Noodles

Ingredients:
¼ (8 oz.) package dried soba noodles
1 tsp. extra virgin olive oil
1 clove garlic, minced
2 tsp. minced fresh ginger
¼ bunch kale, torn into bite-size pieces
Sauce:
3 Tbsp. tahini
2 tsp. rice vinegar
1 ½ tsp. soy sauce
1 ½ tsp. extra virgin olive oil
Drizzle of Sriracha, or other hot sauce
Pinch of ground turmeric (or more, to taste)
2 tsp. water

Directions:

To prepare the sauce, use a medium bowl to combine tahini, rice vinegar, soy sauce, 1 ½ tsp. olive oil, Sriracha, turmeric, and 2 tsp. water. Add more water if needed to get the dressing to your preferred consistency; set aside.

Bring a pot of lightly salted water to a boil. Cook soba noodles at a boil until tender yet firm to the bite, about 5 to 7 minutes. Drain the noodles; set aside

Heat 1 tsp. olive oil in a medium skillet over medium heat. Cook and stir garlic in the olive oil until fragrant, about 1 minute.

Add ginger to the garlic and cook 1 minute more.

Add kale to the skillet; cook and stir for 1 minute more. Reduce heat to low, cover the skillet, and simmer until the kale wilts, about 5 to 10 minutes.

Toss the drained soba noodles in the tahini sauce until coated. Fold the kale into the noodles and sauce and serve.

Nutritional Information

Calories: 178.7

Total Fat: 9.9 g

Saturated Fat: 1.3g

Carbohydrates: 16.9 g

Protein: 5.5 g

Spicy Potato Curry

Ingredients:

1 large potato, peeled and cubed

1 tsp. extra virgin olive oil

1 Tbsp. yellow onion, diced

1 garlic clove, minced

½ tsp. ground cumin

½ tsp. cayenne

¾ tsp. curry powder

¾ tsp. garam masala

2 tsp. fresh ginger root, peeled and minced

Pinch of salt

1 tomato, diced

¼ cup garbanzo beans, rinsed and drained

¼ cup coconut milk

Directions:

Place the cubed potato in a small pot and cover with salted water. Bring to a boil over high heat, then reduce heat to medium-low, cover, and simmer until just tender, about 15 minutes. Drain and allow to steam-dry for a minute or two.

Heat the olive oil in a medium skillet over medium heat. Add the onion and garlic and cook until the onion has softened and turned translucent, about 5 minutes.

Season onion and garlic with with cumin, cayenne pepper, curry powder, garam masala, ginger, and salt; cook for 2 minutes more.

Add the tomatoes, garbanzo beans, and potatoes. Pour in the coconut milk, and bring to a simmer. Simmer 5 to 10 minutes. Place in bowl and serve.

Nutritional Information

Calories: 279.4

Total Fat: 16.2 g

Saturated Fat: 13.1 g
Carbohydrates: 31.4 g
Protein: 2 g

Quinoa Chard Pilaf

Ingredients:

1 tsp. extra virgin olive oil
1 Tbsp. onion, diced
1 clove garlic, minced
¼ cup uncooked quinoa, rinsed
2 Tbsp. canned/prepared lentils, rinsed
½ cup vegetable broth
¼ bunch Swiss chard, stems removed

Directions:

Heat the oil in a small pot over medium heat. Stir in the onion and garlic, and sauté until onion is tender, about 5 minutes.

Add in quinoa and lentils. Pour in the broth. Cover, and cook 15 minutes.

Remove the pot from heat. Shred chard, and gently mix into the pot. Cover, and allow to sit 5 minutes, or until chard is wilted.

Serve and enjoy.

Nutritional Information
Calories: 148.7
Total Fat: 3.1 g
Saturated Fat: 0.6 g

Carbohydrates: 26.6 g

Protein: 3.6 g

Tofu Broccoli Quiche

Ingredients:

1 (9-inch) unbaked vegan pie crust

1 large head of broccoli, chopped

1 Tbsp. olive oil

1 onion, finely chopped

4 cloves garlic, minced

1 pound firm tofu, drained

½ cup soy milk (or preferred milk alternative)

¼ tsp. Dijon mustard

¾ tsp. salt

¼ tsp. ground nutmeg

½ tsp. ground red pepper

Black pepper to taste

1 Tbsp. dried parsley

1/8 cup parmesan flavor soy cheese

Directions:

Preheat oven to 400 degrees F. Bake pie crust in preheated oven for 10 to 12 minutes.

Place broccoli in a steamer over 1 inch of boiling water and cover. Cook until tender but still firm, about 2 to 6 minutes. Drain and set aside.

Heat oil in a large skillet over medium-high heat. Sauté onion and garlic until golden, about 3-5 minutes. Stir in the broccoli and cook for an additional minute.

In a blender, combine tofu, soy milk, mustard, salt, nutmeg, ground red pepper, black pepper, parsley and Parmesan soy cheese and blend until smooth.

In a large bowl combine tofu mixture with broccoli mixture. Pour into pie crust.

Bake in preheated oven until quiche is set, about 35 to 40 minutes. Allow to stand for at least 5 minutes before cutting and serving. Leftovers can be stored in an airtight container in the fridge for up to a week.

Nutritional Information (for $1/6^{th}$ of quiche)

Calories: 353.6

Total Fat: 19.6 g

Saturated Fat: 3.9 g

Carbohydrates: 26.3 g

Protein: 18 g

Lentil and Veggies

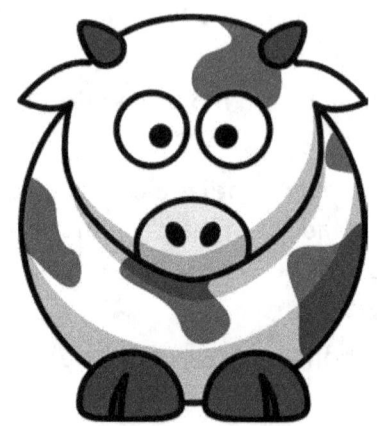

Ingredients:

½ cup long-grain rice, uncooked

2 ½ cups water

1 cup red lentils

1 tsp. olive oil

1 small onion, diced

3 cloves garlic, minced

1 tomato, diced

1/3 cup diced celery

1/3 cup chopped carrots

1/3 cup chopped zucchini

1 (8 oz.) can tomato sauce

1 tsp. dried basil

1 tsp. dried oregano

1 tsp. ground cumin

½ tsp. celery seed

Salt and pepper, to taste

Directions:

Preheat oven to 350 degrees F. In a small bowl, combine basil, oregano, cumin, celery seed, and a pinch of salt and pepper. Set aside.

Place the rice and 1 cup water in a medium pot over high heat and bring to a boil. Cover, reduce heat to low, and simmer 20 minutes.

Place lentils in a pot with the remaining 1 ½ cups water, and bring to a boil. Cook 15 minutes, or until tender.

Heat the oil in a skillet over medium heat, and stir in the onion and garlic. Mix in tomato, celery, carrots, zucchini, and ½ the tomato sauce. Season with ½ the seasoning mix.

In a casserole dish, mix the rice, lentils, and vegetables. Top with remaining tomato sauce, and sprinkle with remaining seasoning.

Bake 30 minutes in the preheated oven, until the top is bubbling. Remove and serve. Store leftovers in an airtight container, in the fridge, for up to a week.

Nutritional Information (for $1/6^{th}$ of bake)

Calories: 192.7

Total Fat: 1.5 g

Saturated Fat: 0.2 g

Carbohydrates: 35.1 g

Protein: 9.7 g

Grilled Tomato-Balsamic Veggies with Couscous

Ingredients:

1 tsp. olive oil

¼ red bell pepper, cut into strips

¼ zucchini, cut into thick slices

¼ small eggplant, cubed

¼ large sweet onion, diced

3 Tbsp. frozen broad beans

2 tomatoes, diced

2 tsp. balsamic vinegar

¼ cup couscous

¼ cup vegetable stock

Directions:

Heat olive oil in a medium grill pan over high heat. When it is very hot, add all the vegetables to the pan. Press down occasionally to get grill lines across them. Turn occasionally to prevent burning. Cook for about 15 minutes, or until the vegetables are evenly browned and cooked through.

Add broad beans to the vegetables. Add diced tomatoes and balsamic vinegar. Simmer for a few minutes while you prepare the couscous.

Place couscous into a medium bowl. Add boiling vegetable stock, and stir with a fork. Cover and allow 2-3 minutes to become softened. Place couscous in a bowl and top with the vegetables.

Nutritional Information

Calories: 82.6
Total Fat: 1.4 g
Saturated Fat: 0.1 g
Carbohydrates: 14.8 g
Protein: 2.7 g

Tempeh Fajitas

Ingredients:
1 ½ tsp. olive oil
¼ (8 oz.) package tempeh, broken into bite-size pieces
2 tsp. soy sauce
1 tsp. lime juice
1 Tbsp. chopped onion
1 clove garlic, minced
1/3 cup chopped green bell pepper
¾ tsp. chopped green chile peppers
1 Tbsp. chopped fresh cilantro
2 corn tortillas

Directions:

Preheat oven to 350 degrees F.

Heat oil in medium skillet over medium heat. Add onion and garlic and cook for 3-5 minutes. Add tempeh with soy sauce and lime juice until tempeh browns.

Add bell peppers, chile peppers, and cilantro and turn heat to medium-high and cook for 5-10 minutes, stirring occasionally.

Meanwhile, heat the corn tortillas in preheated oven until warm and pliable, about 3-5 minutes.

Remove tortillas from oven, fill with tempeh mixture and enjoy.

Nutritional Information
Calories: 154.7
Total Fat: 4.3 g
Saturated Fat: 1.2 g
Carbohydrates: 23.2 g
Protein: 5.8 g

Lentil, Kale, and Red Onion Pasta

Ingredients:
½ cup vegetable broth
2 Tbsp. dry lentils
Pinch of salt
½ bay leaf
1 Tbsp. olive oil
¼ large red onion, chopped
¼ tsp. chopped fresh time
¼ tsp. dried oregano
Salt and pepper, to taste
1 piece vegan sausage, cut into ¼ inch slices (optional)
¼ bunch kale, stems removed and leaves coarsely chopped
1 cup rotini pasta

Directions:

Bring the vegetable broth, lentils, pinch of salt, and bay leaf to a boil in a saucepan over high heat. Reduce heat to medium-low, cover, and cook until the lentils are tender, about 20 minutes. Add additional broth if needed to keep the lentils moist. Discard the bay leaf once done.

As the lentils simmer, heat the olive oil in a skillet over medium-high heat. Stir in the onion, thyme, oregano, salt, and pepper. Cook and stir for 1 minute, then add the sausage. Reduce the heat to medium-low, and cook until the onion has softened, about 10 minutes.

Meanwhile, bring a large pot of lightly salted water to a boil over high heat. Add the kale and rotini pasta. Cook until the rotini is al dente, about 8 minutes. Remove some of the cooking water, and set aside. Drain the pasta, then return to the pot,

Stir in the lentils and onion mixture. Use the reserved cooking liquid to adjust the moistness of the dish to your liking and serve.

Nutritional Information

Calories: 184.5

Total Fat: 4.1 g

Saturated Fat: 0.5 g

Carbohydrates: 27.9 g

Protein: 9 g

Teriyaki Tofu with Pineapple

Ingredients:

¼ (12 oz.) package firm tofu

1/3 cup chopped fresh pineapple

½ cup teriyaki sauce

¼ cup rice (any variety)

½ cup water

Directions:

Cut the tofu into bite-size pieces and place in a baking dish. Add pineapple and pour in teriyaki sauce. Cover and refrigerate for at least 1 hour

Preheat oven to 350 degrees F.

Bake tofu in preheated oven for 20 minutes, or until hot and bubbly.

While the tofu is baking, prepare the rice by placing both the rice and water in a medium saucepan or small pot. Turn the heat to high until it begins to boil, and then reduce to low, cover and let simmer for 15 minutes.

Place rice in a bowl and top with pineapple teriyaki tofu.

Nutritional Information

Calories: 211.5

Total Fat: 1.9 g

Saturated Fat: 0 g

Carbohydrates: 43.1 g

Protein: 5.5 g

Tofu and Red Bell Peppers with Spicy Peanut Sauce

Ingredients:

- 1/2 package (14 oz.) firm or extra-firm tofu
- 1/2 Tbsp. olive oil
- 1/2 Tbsp. soy sauce, divided
- 1/2 medium red bell pepper, seeded, cut into strips
- 1 Tbsp. onion, diced
- 3/4 Tbsp. smooth peanut butter
- 1/2 Tbsp. fresh lime juice
- 2 tsp. Sriracha or other chili-garlic sauce
- 2 tsp. brown sugar
- 3/4 Tbsp. water
- 1/2 Tbsp. cilantro, chopped (optional)

Directions:

Preheat oven to 450 degrees F. Slice tofu into 4 rectangles.

In a shallow bowl, whisk together half the olive oil and half the soy sauce. Dip tofu pieces on all sides to coat.

Brush a baking sheet with a little bit of olive and place tofu pieces on the baking sheet. Scatter peppers and onions around the edges.

Bake 10 minutes; turn tofu, peppers and onions over and continue baking until tofu is golden brown and the vegetables begin to car, about 10-15 minutes more.

In a small saucepan over low heat, whisk together peanut butter, lime juice, chili sauce, brown sugar, water, and remaining soy sauce, until warm.

Remove tofu, peppers, and onion from oven and place in a bowl or on a plate. Drizzle peanut sauce over them and garnish with cilantro.

Nutritional Information

Calories: 275
Total Fat: 11 g
Saturated Fat: 1 g
Carbohydrates: 26.4 g
Protein: 17.6 g

Toasted Almond and Quinoa Salad

Ingredients:

3 Tbsp. slivered almonds

1/4 cup quinoa

1/2 cup water

2 tsp. olive oil

1/2 yellow bell pepper, seeded and cut into 1/2 inch chunks

1 garlic clove, minced

1 scallion, thinly sliced

Pinch of red pepper flakes

1 tsp. chopped fresh thyme

1/2 medium zucchini, cut lengthwise and sliced into 1/2 –inch thick pieces

1/2 large celery stalk, diced

Juice from half a lime

Salt and pepper, to taste

Directions:

Preheat oven to 350 degrees. Place almonds on a baking sheet and toast in the oven until crisp, lightly browned, and fragrant, about 7 minutes. Remove from oven and set aside.

In a medium saucepan, heat 1 tsp. olive oil over medium heat. Add yellow pepper, garlic, scallions, and red-pepper flakes; cook until the pepper is tender, about 5 minutes.

Stir in quinoa, thyme, water, and a pinch of salt. Bring to a boil, reduce to a simmer, cover, and cook 7 minutes.

Stir in zucchini, cover, and cook until quinoa is tender but not mushy, 5 to 8 minutes longer. Remove the saucepan from heat.

Stir in celery, almonds, and remaining tsp. of olive oil. Season with salt and pepper, fluff with a fork. Serve warm or cold and season with a squeeze of lime right before serving.

Nutritional Information
Calories: 277.5
Total Fat: 7.9 g
Saturated Fat: 1 g
Carbohydrates: 43.6 g
Protein: 8 g

Vegan Chili

Ingredients:

2 Tbsp. extra virgin olive oil

1 medium yellow onion, diced

4 garlic cloves, minced

1 1/2 tsp. ground cumin

1 tsp. chili powder

Salt and pepper, to taste

1 medium zucchini, diced into 1/2-inch cubes

3/4 cup tomato paste

1 can (15 oz.) black beans, rinsed and drained

1 can (15 oz.) pinto beans, rinsed and drained

1 can (14 oz.) diced tomatoes with green chiles

1 can (14.5 oz.) diced tomatoes

2 cups water

Directions:

In a large pot, heat oil over medium-high. Add onion and garlic; cook, stirring frequently, until fragrant, about 4 minutes. Add cumin and chili powder, a pinch of salt and pepper, and cook, 1 minute.

Add zucchini and tomato paste; cook, stirring frequently, 3 minutes.

Add in black beans, pinto beans, and both cans diced tomatoes. Add 2 cups water and bring mixture to a boil. Reduce heat to medium, simmer and cook until zucchini is tender and liquid reduces slightly, about 20 minutes. Season with salt and pepper and serve. Extras can be stored in an airtight container, in the fridge, for up to a week.

Nutritional Information (per serving, approximately $1/4^{th}$ of chili)

Calories: 235.5

Total Fat: 3.9 g

Saturated Fat: 0.7 g

Carbohydrates: 41.1 g

Protein: 9 g

One-Pot Marrakesh Stew

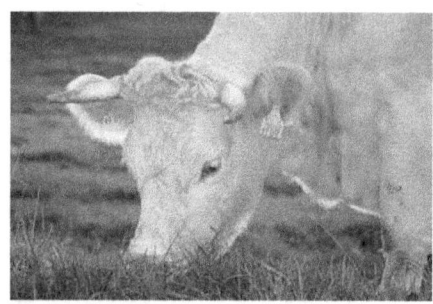

Ingredients:

1 Tbsp. extra-virgin olive oil

1 large red onion, diced

2 tsp ground cumin

1 tsp ground cinnamon

1 tsp ground coriander

3/4 tsp cayenne pepper

1/2 tsp ground allspice

4 large carrots, cut into 1-inch pieces

2 russet potatoes, peeled and cut into 1-inch pieces

1 small butternut squash, peeled, seeded, and cut into 1-inch pieces

Salt and pepper, to taste

1 can (14.5 ounces) diced tomatoes

3 3/4 cups vegetable broth

2 small eggplants, cut into 1-inch pieces

1 can (15.5 ounces) garbanzo beans, rinsed and drained

4 Tbsp. couscous

1/3 cup boiled water

Directions:

Place the couscous in a large bowl and add 1/3 cup boiled water. Stir, cover tightly and let stand for 10 minutes.

In an 8-quart Dutch oven or heavy pot, heat oil over medium-high. Add onion and cook, stirring occasionally, until soft, 5 minutes.

Add cumin, cinnamon, coriander, cayenne, and allspice and cook until fragrant, 1 minute.

Add carrots, potatoes, and squash and season with salt and pepper. Cook, stirring occasionally, until beginning to brown, 5 minutes. Add tomatoes and broth—be sure vegetables are completely covered. If not, add water. Bring to a gentle simmer and cook, uncovered, 20 minutes.

Add eggplant, stir to combine, and simmer until eggplant is tender, about 20 minutes more. Stir in chickpeas, season to taste with salt and pepper, and cook until garbanzo beans are warmed through, 3 to 5 minutes.

Serve stew with couscous. Leftovers can be stored in an airtight container, in the fridge for up to a week, or frozen, for up to a month.

Nutritional Information (for one serving, approx. 1/6th of stew, with couscous)

Calories: 234.3

Total Fat: 5.9 g

Saturated Fat: 0.3 g

Carbohydrates: 41 g

Protein: 4.3 g

Crispy Sesame Tofu and Broccoli

Ingredients:

1/2 block firm tofu

1 Tbsp. sesame seeds

1/4 Tbsp. sesame oil

3/4 Tbsp. soy sauce

1 cup broccoli, cut into 1/2 inch pieces

2 Tbsp. water

Salt and pepper, to taste

Directions:

Slice tofu lengthwise into 2 equal pieces, then down the middle to make 4 squares. Pat squares dry with a paper towel, pressing to help remove more liquid if needed.

Spread the sesame seeds on a plate. Press both sides of each tofu square into sesame seeds. In a large nonstick skillet, heat sesame oil over medium heat. Cook tofu, until golden brown, 4 to 6 minutes per side.

Add the soy sauce and continue cooking and turning the tofu, until it has absorbed all the liquid, about 1 minute. Remove from pan and set aside.

Add broccoli, 2 Tbsp. water, and a pinch of salt and pepper to skillet. Simmer, covered, until broccoli is tender, about 5 minutes.

Place broccoli and tofu on a plate, drizzle with additional sesame oil, if desired and serve.

Nutritional Information

Calories: 148
Total Fat: 5 g
Saturated Fat: 1.8 g
Carbohydrates: 18 g
Protein: 14 g

Stuffed Sweet Potatoes

Ingredients:

1 large round sweet potato

1/4 Tbsp. olive oil

1/4 small onion, chopped

1 garlic clove, minced

1/2 tsp. finely chopped rosemary

Pinch of crushed red pepper flakes

Salt and pepper, to taste

1 cup kale, trimmed and thinly sliced

1/8 (14 oz. package) firm tofu, cut into 1/2 –inch cubes

2 Tbsp. water

Directions:

Preheat oven to 375 degrees F. Line a rimmed baking sheet with parchment paper. Bake sweet potato on sheet until tender but not completely cooked through, 55 minutes to 1 hour. Leave oven on.

Once the potato is cool enough to handle, cut off the top quarter and discard. Scoop out and reserve flesh, leaving a 1/2-inch-thick shell; set shells aside. Coarsely chop the flesh; set aside.

Heat oil in a large nonstick skillet over medium-high heat. Add onion, garlic, rosemary, salt, and red pepper flakes; cook, stirring occasionally, about 3 minutes. Add kale; cook, stirring occasionally, until kale has wilted, about 5 minutes. Stir in reserved chopped sweet potatoes, the tofu, and water. Cook for an additional minute.

Place sweet potato shell on a baking sheet. Spoon filling into shell and cover with foil. Bake until heated through, about 30 minutes. Serve

Nutritional Information
Calories: 190.5
Total Fat: 4.5 g
Saturated Fat: 0.6 g
Carbohydrates: 32 g
Protein: 5.5 g

Tofu Kebabs with Cilantro Dressing

Ingredients:
1/2 cup fresh cilantro
1 Tbsp. olive oil
1/4 small jalapeno, seeded
1 tsp. grated fresh ginger
1/2 Tbsp. fresh lime juice
1 scallion, white and green parts separated and cut into 1-inch lengths
Salt and pepper, to taste
1/2 package (14 oz.) extra-firm tofu, cut into 3-4 pieces

1/2 summer squash, cut into 1-inch pieces

Directions:

Heat grill to medium. In a food processor, combine cilantro, oil, jalapeno, ginger, lime juice, and scallion greens. Blend until smooth; season with salt and pepper.

In a bowl, combine tofu, scallion whites, and a drizzle of olive oil; season with salt and pepper. Thread tofu and scallion whites onto 1 skewer, and then thread squash onto 1 skewer.

Clean and lightly oil hot grates. Grill squash kebab, covered, until tender, 11 to 13 minutes, turning occasionally. Grill tofu kebab until scallions are soft, about 4 to 6 minutes, turning occasionally.

Brush both with cilantro sauce and grill 30 seconds more. Serve kebabs with remaining cilantro sauce.

Nutritional Information

Calories: 254

Total Fat: 10 g

Saturated Fat: 1 g

Carbohydrates: 27 g

Protein:14 g

Four-Grain Vegan Salad

Ingredients:

¼ cup amaranth seeds

¼ cup vegetable broth

¼ cup quinoa

½ cup vegetable broth

¼ cup millet

½ cup vegetable broth

¼ cup cooked brown basmati or jasmine rice

¼ tsp. grated orange zest

¼ cup fresh orange segments

¼ cup diced fennel

¼ cup diced radishes

1 Tbsp. olive oil

2 Tbsp. fresh orange juice

½ Tbsp. red wine vinegar

¼ Tbsp. chopped fresh fennel fronds

Pinch fresh dill

Salt and Pepper, to taste

Directions:

To cook the amaranth—place a small saucepan over medium high heat, add the amaranth. Toast for 4-5 minutes. While amaranth is cooking, bring ¼ cup broth to boil in a medium saucepan. Add amaranth and a pinch of salt to the broth and cover; reduce the heat to simmer for 7 minutes. Remove from heat and set aside.

To cook the quinoa—Bring ½ cup vegetable broth and pinch of salt and pepper to a boil in a medium saucepan. Add the quinoa, cover the pan and reduce the heat. Simmer until liquid has been absorbed, about 7-12 minutes. Set aside.

To cook the millet-- place a small saucepan over medium high heat, add the millet. Toast for 4-5 minutes. Remove pan from heat, pour millet into a bowl and add cold water. Swirl and drain. Bring ¼ cup broth to boil in a medium saucepan. Add millet and a pinch of salt to the broth and cover; reduce the heat to simmer for 15 minutes. Remove from heat and set aside.

Combine all the prepared ingredients in a large bowl. Refrigerate, covered, for at least 1 hour or as long as 3 to 4 days before serving.

Remove from the refrigerator and serve at room temperature.

Nutritional Information

Calories: 379

Total Fat: 7 g

Saturated Fat: 1.9 g

Carbohydrates: 68 g

Protein:11 g

Barley with Winter Greens Pesto

Ingredients:

½ cup hulled barley

¾ cup water

½ bunch Swiss Chard, stems removed

½ bunch mustard greens, stems removed

2 Tbsp. almonds, toasted

1 ½ tsp. sherry vinegar

1 garlic clove, minced

1 ½ Tbsp. walnut oil

Salt and pepper

Directions:

Place the barley, a pinch of salt, and water in a medium saucepan. Bring to a boil over high heat, and then reduce the heat to low and simmer, covered, until the barley is tender but still slightly chewy, about 30 to 45 minutes. Drain and set aside to cool.

Bring a medium saucepan of salted water to a boil over high heat. Add the chard and mustard greens and blanch for 1 minute or until wilted and tender. Drain and let cool slightly.

Place the cooled greens, almonds, vinegar, and garlic in a food processor. Add the walnut oil in a steady stream until all of the ingredients are evenly incorporated, about 2 minutes. Scrape down the sides of the bowl, season with salt and pepper, and process until smooth.

Place the reserved barley in a large bowl, add the pesto, and mix to combine. Season with salt and pepper and serve.

Nutritional Information
Calories: 314
Total Fat: 14 g
Saturated Fat: 1 g
Carbohydrates: 37 g
Protein:10 g

Cajun Style Tempeh Po' Boy

Ingredients:
½ (8 oz.) package tempeh, sliced horizontally into ½-inch pieces
2 Tbsp. olive oil
¼ large yellow onion, thinly sliced
½ tsp. garlic powder
½ tsp. paprika
½ tsp. chili powder
Pinch red chili flakes
Pinch cayenne pepper

½ tsp. dried thyme

½ tsp. dried oregano

Salt and pepper

½ large green bell pepper, seeds removed, cut into long ¼-inch wide strips

½ cup water

2 Tbsp. tomato paste

Drizzle pure maple syrup

Drizzle balsamic vinegar

2 tomatoes, diced

Whole wheat bread roll (or preferred bread)

Directions:

Preheat oven to 350°F.

In a medium bowl combine the tempeh pieces with a 1/2 Tbsp. of the olive oil and toss well.

Heat 1 ½ Tbsp. of the olive oil in a medium skillet over medium-high heat. Add the tempeh fingers and cook for 5 to 7 minutes, adding more oil if necessary, until lightly browned. Turn the fingers over and cook for 5 to 7 minutes more, until lightly browned on the other side. Transfer the tempeh to a large plate lined with paper towels.

Combine ½ Tbsp. of the olive oil with the onion, garlic powder, paprika, chili powder, red chili flakes, cayenne, thyme, oregano, pinch of salt and pepper in a large nonstick skillet over medium-low heat. Slowly sauté for 15 minutes, stirring often to prevent burning, until well caramelized.

Add the green bell peppers to the skillet, and sauté for 10 more minutes, or until the bell peppers are softened.

In a large bowl combine ½ cup water, tomato paste, maple syrup, vinegar, and a pinch of salt. Whisk well. Add the diced tomatoes with their juices and onion and green pepper mixture. Stir well.

Place the tempeh in a small casserole dish. Pour the sauce on top, covering all the tempeh fingers.

Cover the dish with foil and bake for 45 minutes, or until most of the sauce is absorbed.

Cut bread roll open, if needed. Place tempeh pieces on one slice, making sure you cover it with plenty of sauce, and place another slice on top

Nutritional Information

Calories: 356

Total Fat: 12 g

Saturated Fat: 1 g

Carbohydrates: 42 g

Protein: 20g

Celery Root Soup

Ingredients:

3 Tbsp. extra-virgin olive oil

1 cup thinly sliced, white and light green parts only

3 medium celery root, (also known as celeriac), peeled and cut into 1-inch chunks

2 large Yukon Gold potatoes, peeled and cut into 1-inch chunks

1 Granny Smith apple (or other tart variety), peeled, cored, and cut into 1-inch chunks

2 garlic cloves, peeled and smashed

2 tsp. salt, plus more as needed

black pepper

3 cups water

2 cups vegetable broth

Directions:

Heat oil in a large saucepan with a tightfitting lid over medium-high heat until shimmering.

Add leek and cook, stirring occasionally, until softened and translucent, about 3 minutes. Add celery root, potatoes, apple, garlic, salt, and a pinch of pepper. Stir to coat vegetables with oil.

Add water and broth, and bring to a boil. Cover, reduce heat to low, and simmer until vegetables just give way when pierced with a knife, about 20 to 25 minutes.

Remove 1 cup of liquid from the saucepan; set aside. Using a blender, purée the soup in batches until smooth, removing the small cap from the blender lid and covering the space with a kitchen towel (this allows steam from the hot soup to escape and prevents the blender lid from popping off).

Once blended, transfer the soup back to the saucepan and keep warm over low heat. If the soup is too thick, add the reserved liquid a little at a time until the soup reaches the desired consistency.

Taste and season with additional salt and pepper as needed and serve. Leftover soup can be stored in an airtight container, in the fridge, for up to a week.

Nutritional Information (per serving, 1/4th of soup)

Calories: 151

Total Fat: 4.2 g

Saturated Fat: 0.1 g

Carbohydrates: 27 g

Protein:1.3 g

Garbanzo Cakes with Mashed Avocado

Ingredients:

¼ cup bulgur wheat

1 cup water

¼ cup loosely packed parsley leaves

¼ cup loosely packed mint leaves

¼ cup loosely packed cilantro leaves

1 medium clove garlic, roughly chopped

¼ teaspoon ground coriander

½ serrano or jalapeño chili, stemmed, seeded, and roughly chopped

½ can (15 ounce) can of garbanzo beans, drained and rinsed

Salt and Pepper

¼ cup flour

¼ cup water

¾ vegan panko-style breadcrumbs

¼ cup olive oil

½ avocado

½ Tbsp. lime juice

Directions:

Bring 1 cup of water to a boil over high heat. Add bulgur wheat and cook until tender, about 10 minutes. Drain carefully.

While wheat cooks, combine parsley, mint, cilantro, garlic, jalapeño and coriander in a food processor. Pulse until finely chopped, scraping down sides as necessary, about 10 to 12 short pulses. Add half garbanzo beans and pulse until a rough puree is formed, scraping down sides as necessary, about 8 to 10 short pulses. Transfer to a bowl.

Add remaining chickpeas to food processor and pulse until roughly chopped, 4 to 6 pulses. Transfer to bowl with chickpea/herb mixture. When bulgur wheat has drained, add to bowl. Season with salt and pepper, then fold mixture together, starting with a rubber spatula, and finishing by hand when cool enough to handle. Form mixture into patties roughly 3/4-inch thick and 3 inches wide (you should be able to make 2-3 patties)

Combine flour and water in a medium bowl and whisk until smooth. Place breadcrumbs in a second bowl.

Working one patty at a time, dip in flour mixture to coat, then transfer to breadcrumbs. Cover with breadcrumbs on all sides, and transfer to a plate. Repeat with remaining patties.

Put half of oil in a large cast iron or non-stick skillet over medium-high heat until shimmering. Add the patties in a single layer and cook, swirling pan occasionally, until golden brown on bottoms, about 2 minutes. Carefully flip and cook second side, swirling pan occasionally as they cook, about 2 minutes longer.

Place avocado in a small bowl and mash the flesh with a fork. Season with salt and add lime juice. Serve fried chickpea patties with mashed avocado, sliced onions, herbs, and lime or lemon wedges.

Nutritional Information

Calories: 696.8

Total Fat: 28 g

Saturated Fat: 4 g

Carbohydrates: 96 .2 g

Protein: 15 g

Vegan Paella

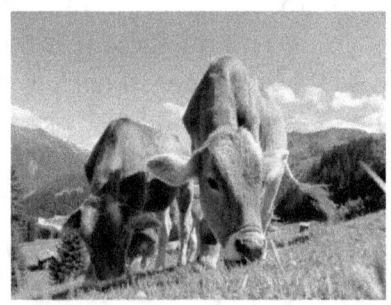

Ingredients:

1/2 cup boiling water

¼ cup white rice

¾ tsp. olive oil

¼ onion, chopped

1 garlic clove, minced

¼ green bell pepper, sliced

¼ red bell pepper, sliced

½ tomato, diced

½ cup vegetable broth

1 tsp. paprika

½ tsp. ground turmeric

¼ cup peas

¼ cup drained and quartered canned artichoke hearts

Salt and pepper

Directions:

Mix boiling water and rice together in a bowl; let stand for 20 minutes. Drain.

Heat olive oil in a large skillet over medium heat; cook and stir onion and garlic until onion is transparent, about 5 minutes. Add green bell pepper, red bell pepper, and tomato; cook and stir until peppers are slightly tender, about 3 minutes.

Mix rice and vegetable broth into onion-pepper mixture; bring to a boil. Reduce heat to low and simmer. Add paprika, turmeric and a pinch of salt and pepper; cover skillet and simmer until rice is tender, about 20 minutes.

Stir peas and artichoke hearts into rice mixture and cook until heated through, about 1 minute more. Serve hot.

Nutritional Information

Calories: 124.8

Total Fat: 1.6g

Saturated Fat: 0.2 g

Carbohydrates: 25.5 g

Protein: 2.1g

Spicy Quinoa with Edamame

Ingredients:

¾ cup water

½ cup quinoa

1 tsp. vegetable bouillon

¾ cup shelled edamame

1 tsp. olive oil

½ sweet onion, diced

½ bell pepper, diced

1 ½ tsp. minced fresh ginger

2 garlic cloves, minced

1 Tbsp. soy sauce

2 tsp. chopped fresh cilantro

1 tsp. Sriracha, or other hot chili paste

Directions:

Bring water, quinoa, and vegetable bouillon to a boil in a medium pot; stir in edamame, cover, and simmer until quinoa is tender, 15 to 20 minutes.

Heat olive oil in a medium skillet over medium heat; cook and stir onions and bell peppers until onions are translucent, about 5 minutes.

Add ginger and garlic; cook and stir until fragrant, about 2 minutes. Remove from heat; stir in soy sauce, cilantro, and chili paste.

Combine onion mixture and quinoa mixture; simmer, stirring occasionally, until excess broth has been absorbed, about 5 minutes. Serve.

Nutritional Information

Calories: 165.8
Total Fat: 5 g
Saturated Fat: 0.6 g
Carbohydrates: 21.4 g
Protein: 8.8 g

Avocado Pasta with Blackened Veggies

Ingredients:

Veggies:

¼ head broccoli, cut into 1-inch florets

½ red bell pepper, cut into ½ inch chunks

¼ yellow onion, thinly sliced into rings

2 tsp. olive oil

Juice from half a lime

Pinch of salt

Sauce:

1 avocado, peeled and chopped

Juice from ½ lime

1 garlic clove, peeled

2 Tbsp. chopped fresh cilantro

Salt and pepper

Pasta:

1 ½ cup penne pasta

Pinch of salt

Directions:

Preheat oven to 450 degrees F.

Combine broccoli, red bell peppers, and yellow onion in a large bowl. Add olive oil, juice from ½ a lime, and a pinch of salt; toss to coat. Spread vegetables onto a baking sheet.

Roast vegetables for 30 minutes, stirring 1 or 2 times, until edges begin to blacken. Remove from oven and cool slightly.

Fill a large pot with water and a pinch of salt; bring to a boil. Stir in penne and return to a boil. Cook pasta uncovered, stirring occasionally, until cooked through but still firm to the bite, about 11 minutes; drain.

Blend avocado, juice from ½ a lime, garlic, and pinch of salt and pepper in a food processor or blender until sauce is smooth, scraping down sides as needed. Add chopped cilantro and pulse until just incorporated.

Gently toss pasta, roasted vegetables, and sauce together in a bowl. Serve.

Nutritional Information

Calories: 326.7

Total Fat: 11.5 g

Saturated Fat: 1.2 g

Carbohydrates: 45.6 g

Protein: 10.2 g

Black-eyed Peas with Collard Greens and Turnips

Ingredients:

¼ cup brown rice

½ cup water

½ cup dried black-eye peas

1 cup water, or as needed to cover peas

1 tsp. soy margarine

½ turnip, peeled and chopped

¼ bunch collard greens, chopped

Salt and pepper

1 garlic clove, minced

1 tomato, chopped

1 tsp. balsamic vinaigrette salad dressing

1 tsp olive oil (optional)

Directions:

Place black-eyed peas into a medium container and cover with several inches of cool water; let stand 8 hours to overnight. Drain and rinse.

Prepare the rice by placing both the rice and ½ cup water in a medium saucepan or small pot. Turn the heat to high until it begins to boil, and then reduce to low, cover and let simmer for 15 minutes.

In a small pot, cover black-eyed peas with fresh water. Bring to a boil over high heat, then reduce the heat to medium-low; cover and simmer until peas are tender, 40 to 60 minutes. Drain.

Heat soy margarine in a skillet over medium heat. Add turnip and collard greens a pinch of salt and pepper; cook for 2 minutes.

Stir black-eyed peas, garlic, and tomatoes into collard mixture; cook and stir until collards are tender, about 5 minutes.

Season with balsamic vinaigrette and olive oil and serve.

Nutritional Information

Calories: 159

Total Fat: 2.6 g
Saturated Fat: 0.3 g
Carbohydrates: 30.9 g
Protein: 3 g

Vegan Black Bean Quesadillas

Ingredients:

¼ (15 oz.) can great Northern beans, drained and rinsed

4 Tbsp. diced tomatoes

1 clove garlic, minced

½ tsp. ground cumin

Pinch of chili powder

Pinch cayenne pepper

¼ cup black beans, drained and rinsed

Pinch of salt

2 whole grain tortillas

1 Tbsp. fresh, chopped cilantro

1 tsp. olive oil

Directions:

Blend great Northern beans, 3 Tbsp. tomatoes, and garlic in a food processor until smooth; add cumin, chili powder, pinch of salt and cayenne and blend again.

Transfer bean mixture to a bowl. Stir black beans, 1 Tbsp. tomatoes, and cilantro into bean mixture.

Heat oil in skillet over medium-high heat. Place a tortilla in the hot oil. Spread about bean filling onto the tortilla.

Place another tortilla on top of filling; cook until filling is warmed, about 10 minutes.

Flip quesadilla to cook the second side until lightly browned, 3 to 5 minutes.

Nutritional Information

Calories: 121.9

Total Fat: 1.5 g

Saturated Fat: 0.3 g

Carbohydrates: 21.4 g

Protein: 5.7 g

Stuffed Red Bell Pepper

Ingredients:

¼ cup brown rice

½ cup water

1 red bell pepper, top and seeds removed

1 tsp olive oil

¼ onion, chopped

1 garlic clove, chopped

¼ (15 oz.) can black-eyed peas, rinsed and drained

1 large Swiss Chard leaf, chopped

Salt and pepper, to taste

Directions:

Preheat oven to 350 degrees F. Spray a baking sheet with cooking spray.

Bring the brown rice and water to a boil in a saucepan over high heat. Reduce the heat to medium-low, cover, and simmer until the rice is tender and the liquid has been absorbed, 15-30 minutes.

Place the red pepper on the prepared baking sheet, and bake until tender, about 15 minutes.

Heat the olive oil in a skillet over medium heat, cook and stir the onion and garlic until the onion is translucent, about 5 minutes.

Stir in the black-eyed peas and chard. Bring the mixture to a simmer, and cook until the chard is wilted, 5 to 8 minutes. Mix in the cooked brown rice, sprinkle with salt and pepper to taste, and lightly stuff the mixture into the red pepper. Serve hot.

Nutritional Information
Calories: 100
Total Fat: 0.8 g
Saturated Fat: 0.1 g
Carbohydrates: 20.8 g
Protein: 2.4 g

Couscous with Olives and Sun-dried Tomatoes

Ingredients:
½ cup vegetable broth, divided
¼ cup water
½ cup pearl couscous
Pinch salt and pepper

1 Tbsp. and 1 tsp olive oil, divided

2 Tbsp. pine nuts

1 clove garlic, minced

¼ shallot, minced

2 Tbsp. sliced black olives

1 Tbsp. sun- dried tomatoes packed in oil, drained and chopped

1 Tbsp. chopped fresh parsley

Directions:

Bring ¼ cup vegetable broth and water to a boil in a saucepan, stir in couscous, and mix in salt and black pepper. Reduce heat to low and simmer until liquid is absorbed, about 8 minutes.

Heat 1 tsp. olive oil in a skillet over medium-high heat; stir in pine nuts and cook, stirring frequently, until pine nuts smell toasted and are golden brown, about 1 minute. Remove from heat.

Heat remaining 1 Tbsp. olive oil in a saucepan; cook and stir garlic and shallot in the hot oil until softened, about 2 minutes. Stir black olives and sun-dried tomatoes into garlic mixture and cook until heated through, 2 to 3 minutes, stirring often.

Slowly pour in remaining vegetable broth and bring mixture to a boil. Reduce heat to low and simmer until sauce has reduced, 8 to 10 minutes.

Transfer couscous to a bowl, mix with sauce, and serve topped with parsley and pine nuts.

Nutritional Information

Calories: 142.1

Total Fat: 7.3 g

Saturated Fat: 1 g

Carbohydrates: 15.8 g

Protein: 3.3 g

Braised White Beans and Chard

Ingredients:

¼ bunch Swiss chard

1 Tbsp. olive oil

¼ medium yellow onion, diced

1 garlic clove, minced

Salt and pepper

½ (15 oz.) can cannellini beans, drained and rinsed

½ cup vegetable broth

1 Tbsp. coarsely chopped fresh parsley

1 tsp. white wine vinegar

Directions:

Trim the ends from the chard stems and discard. Cut off the stems at the base of the leaves and slice crosswise into 1/4-inch pieces; set aside. Stack the leaves and cut them into bite-size pieces; set aside.

Heat the oil in a Dutch oven or a heavy-bottomed pot over medium heat until shimmering. Add the chard stems, onion, and garlic and season with salt and pepper. Cook, stirring occasionally, until the vegetables have softened, about 8 minutes.

Add the chard leaves, beans, broth, and pinch of salt. Cook, stirring occasionally, until the leaves are wilted and the mixture has come to a simmer. Continue to simmer, stirring occasionally, until the chard is tender and the broth has thickened slightly, about 5 minutes more.

Remove from the heat and stir in the parsley and vinegar. Taste and season with salt and pepper as needed.

Nutritional Information

Calories: 185

Total Fat: 9 g

Saturated Fat: 1.9 g

Carbohydrates: 21 g

Protein: 5 g

Miso Soup with Napa Cabbage

Ingredients:

1 tsp. olive oil

¼ medium yellow onion, thinly sliced

1 tsp. peeled, and finely chopped fresh ginger

1 garlic clove, minced

1 ½ cups vegetable broth

½ Tbsp. soy sauce

½ (12 oz.) package Udon Noodles

¼ medium napa cabbage, cored, halved lengthwise and cut into 1 inch pieces

½ carrot, julienned

¼ cup white miso

Sriracha, or other chili sauce, for serving

Directions:

Bring a medium pot of heavily salted water to a boil over medium-high heat.

Add the udon to the pot of boiling water and cook according to the package directions. Drain in a colander and, while stirring, rinse the noodles with cold water until they're cooled and no longer sticky. Put the noodles in a deep bowl.

Meanwhile, heat the oil in a medium saucepan over medium heat until shimmering. Add the onion, ginger, garlic, and carrot, and cook, stirring occasionally, until the onions have softened, about 5 minutes.

Increase the heat to medium high. Add the broth and soy sauce and stir to combine.

Add the cabbage to the pan, stir to combine, and simmer until the cabbage is tender, about 5 minutes. Add the miso and stir to combine. Taste and season with salt as needed.

Top udon noodles with cabbage mixture and hot sauce, if desired.

Nutritional Information

Calories: 130.9

Total Fat: 2.1 g

Saturated Fat: 0g

Carbohydrates: 24g

Protein: 4 g

www.ingramcontent.com/pod-product-compliance
Lightning Source LLC
Chambersburg PA
CBHW071436070526
44578CB00001B/99